Healthy Eating Healthy Living

Healthy YOU

Samadhi Artemisa, A.P.

Art Director, Cover Design, Interior Layout and Design:
Matt D. Smith (www.MDSmithDesign.com)

Interior Layout:
Martin Murphy

Editing:
Jill Anderson
Patricia Charpentier (www.WritingYourLife.org)
Eileen Glaser
Mary Jones
Amy Moore, N.D., D.O.M., A.P.
Jennifer Taylor, Ph.D.

Photography:
All photos were taken by Samadhi Artemisa, A.P. except:
Randy Badilo: page 106
Michael Cairns (www.MichaelCairns.com): back cover and pages 9, 11,
13, 31, 35, 36, 45, 155
Laura Croson: page 141
Fran Diehl: page 72

Your Guide to

— *Reclaim* —

YOUR VITALITY
GET HEALTHY

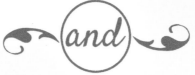

(and)

FEEL GREAT!

Samadhi Artemisa

Table
of
Contents

Section 1

Healthy Living: Using Holistic Home Remedies and Knowing When to Get Help 1

Section 2

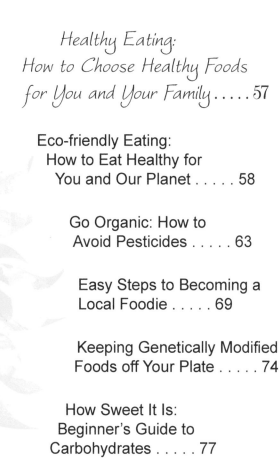

Section 3

Healthy Eating:
How to Choose Healthy Foods
for You and Your Family 57

Section 4

Nutrition and Food:
Your Indispensable Guide
to Selecting and Storing
Fruits, Vegetables
and Nuts 89

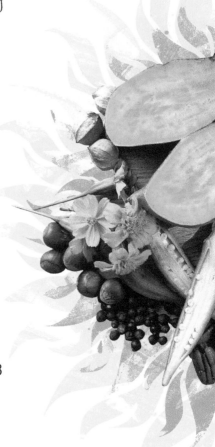

How to Select,
Store and Enjoy Fruits

Section 4 *(continued)*

Section 5

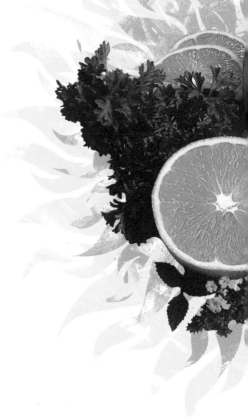

Section 5 (continued)

Section 5 (continued)

Healthy Beverages for Every Mood: Teas, Cleansers and Tonics

Section 5 (continued)

**Bonus: More Great Recipes—
Just Too Good to Leave Out**

Preface

By Ellen Tart-Jensen, Ph.D., D.Sc., C.C.I.I.
Author of: Health Is Your Birthright:
How to Create the Health You Deserve

There comes a time in every person's life when they begin to understand who they are, what they believe in and how they choose to live their lives. As a practicing acupuncturist and iridologist, Samadhi Artemisa has done just that. She has chosen to follow the "natural path."

Several years ago, I had the opportunity to get to know Samadhi as her instructor at a university where she was studying natural health. She was an ardent student who worked hard to do her best. Some of the books she studied included those written by my late father-in-law, Dr. Bernard Jensen, Ph.D., D.C., N.D. He was a pioneer for sixty years teaching good nutrition, cleansing, and proper care of the soil in over 50 different countries worldwide. During that time, I had the opportunity to work with him at his Hidden Valley Health Ranch and saw people with the worst health conditions get well by cleansing, juicing, and eating fresh fruits and vegetables grown on the land. Dr. Jensen always said, "Nature will heal when given the opportunity."

In my own natural health practice, I have seen the research of Dr. Bernard Jensen proven time and again. When people begin to live in rhythm and harmony with nature, eat organically grown foods, drink pure water, cleanse, exercise and think happy thoughts, their lives change for the better. Aches and pains disappear and they begin to feel happy and alive again.

Samadhi lives, practices and teaches what she so fervently believes. In this wonderful collection of articles, she has graciously shared with the world some of her own vital health secrets as well as how to be a good steward of the earth. She teaches the importance of choice in selecting foods best for you that were grown sustainably without chemicals, sprays and pesticides. As you read, you will learn which foods are the most heavily sprayed, and which foods are not. Important information about genetically modified foods (GMO's) and the destruction these cause to our bodies and to our planet will be revealed. Throughout these pages, the reader can virtually feel the presence of Samadhi's passion shining through each refreshing word as she teaches how to eat and live for optimal wellness.

Prepare to be inspired as you journey with this uplifting author through her amazing organic garden, where you will learn about the seasons of fruits and vegetables. She will teach you the importance of eating organically grown foods in order to conserve our Earth's resources. You will learn the value of eating a variety of foods with all of the rainbow colors in order to get the nutrients you need for health. Learn how to use the bitter greens and red beets as digestive tonics and liver cleansers. If you have a sweet tooth, you will learn about some very sweet fruits that will leave you feeling satisfied while also providing you with rich nutrients and antioxidants.

Throughout this book, you will learn the health values of many different fruits, vegetables, nuts and seeds and how to best prepare and store them. You will enjoy delicious recipes that leave you feeling energized, alert and vibrant. You will cleanse and strengthen your body with joy and ease, drinking delicious smoothies, and eating satisfying soups and crunchy salads. These foods will help improve digestion and prevent constipation. If you would like to become slim and tone your body, you will learn the secrets to achieving your ideal weight.

In addition to all of the information about foods, you will learn many other tools for great health including acupuncture, skin brushing and iridology. You will learn valuable remedies for a wide variety of ailments such as insomnia, pain, sinus congestion, hormone imbalances, arthritis, asthma, depression, anxiety, addictions, problems with fertility and pregnancy-related symptoms.

Finally, you will learn about metamorphosis and how to become a new you. Samadhi takes you through an amazing analogy of the human life and the many stages of changing like a caterpillar into a butterfly. So if you are ready to let go of the old, make room for the new and learn to fly, this book will take you on that transformational journey!

Introduction

By Samadhi Artemisa, A.P.

There is not one right food, diet or supplement for everyone. Foods that benefit your body may not taste good and foods that taste good may have a negative effect on your health. Foods that are favorable during childhood, adolescence, pregnancy, athletic training or into your elder years may not always be good for you, right for your spouse, your family or your neighbor. We all have unique nutritional needs at different times in life and there are numerous paths to wellness. I prefer the holistic path that empowers each person as an individual.

By my definition, holistic living is about personal accountability, self awareness and daily choices. It is about prevention, with emphasis on building up the body before it breaks down from stress, lack of nutrition, indulgent lifestyle, lack of exercise, lack of sleep or overwork. Through my training and clinical experience, I understand that nutrient deficiencies can take months or years to become noticeable physical symptoms, and that physical symptoms may never develop into a disease.

Some people think if they take a multivitamin it will make up for eating junk food. They prefer to take a pill rather than adjust their diet, habits or way of thinking. There are emotional, social, economic, genetic and cultural reasons for each of our choices. Overnight changes to habitual patterns can sometimes feel overwhelming, be difficult to make and a struggle to commit to.

Many clients come to see me after exhaustive medical testing, medications, second, third and fourth opinions that yield no relief and result in complete frustration with Western medicine. A holistic approach can provide the missing pieces along the journey to wellness. Holistic healthcare puts the responsibility back on the individual, offering ways to balance the lifestyle and diet, which is different then the Western approach of medications, testing and surgeries. There is an appropriate time and place for both allopathic and holistic healthcare.

In my childhood, I overcame many health challenges by changing my diet. I am fortunate that my parents took me for food allergy testing at age four. After eliminating dairy products, corn, food additives, chocolate and more things than I would have liked, many of my symptoms subsided. At the age of twelve, I had a roller skating mishap that triggered a hereditary kidney weakness, leading to reconstructive kidney surgery and many years of follow-up procedures and monitoring. Through these experiences, I learned that I have to take extra care of my digestive tract and urinary system. I now understand that this is what inspired me early in life: the basic idea that there were things I could do to influence my recovery and my health.

In my late teens, I worked in a health food store, started exploring a vegetarian diet, vegan and Indian cooking and began practicing yoga. I have been exploring nutrition, food, all different styles of food preparation, supplements, cleansing, juicing, fasting, exercising, alternative therapies and the effects they have on the mind, body and the environment for my entire adult life.

After 25 years of trying to define myself as an experimental vegan, vegetarian, raw foodie, flexitarian and occasional meat eater, I have finally come to realize that I don't need to define myself socially in these ways anymore. I accept that nature provides us with many bounties—a cornucopia of all different colors, seasons and types of foods. There is absolutely no substitute for fresh, nutritious food, exercise, time in nature, time for rest and play, a happy, peaceful mindset and a good night's sleep.

Many of my health challenges have been easily resolved with an herb, a food or a simple lifestyle change. Other conditions have taken 10 or 15 years to finally shift as the layers peel away and I find balance physically, emotionally and energetically. Just as it can take years for deficiencies to develop, it can also take years to recover from physical and emotional trauma. It can also take years to understand and implement what healthy living is for you as an individual.

Some people think just buying organic food, going gluten-free or eating a salad is going to fix everything. It is always nice when simple changes quickly yield noticeable results. However, even with dramatic changes in diet and lifestyle, sometimes genetic deficiencies, stress from a strained relationship or difficult work environment can be the reason the body takes time to heal.

Many people become impatient after applying only a small effort and give up. Be patient on your path to wellness. Home-cooked meals may not fit into your schedule right now, organic food may seem too expensive and visiting a farm may seem impossible because you live in a big city. Just take what you can from what I offer here and do the best you can with the time, energy and resources you have.

I have the tremendous honor to share my knowledge with my clients, students and, now, with you through my writing. I emphasize a holistic perspective, embracing the importance of food, daily habits and how individual health is linked to the health of our environment. When I am asked what I like about my work my response is, "Helping people be healthy." I am so deeply rewarded seeing the joy on my clients' faces when they tell me they successfully lost weight after years of yo-yo dieting, that they are finally sleeping through the night because of the care they received from me or that they finally have relief from digestive issues, menopausal symptoms or skin conditions when no other practitioner could help them.

Holistic healthcare is something I provide for my clients; I offer a sampling of my wellness tips for you in this book. I have a monthly column in "A Better You" of the *Orlando Sentinel* newspaper. This book is a compilation of some of my published articles from the last few years. It is not intended to be a comprehensive encyclopedia on any one subject; rather it is a detailed introduction to help you get started with healthy eating and healthy living.

This book also marks my debut as a photographer. All the images are my creations unless otherwise noted in the opening credits. I am excited to share my love of food and nature with you through my writing and photos. I hope to inspire you to choose wholesome, organic foods, shop at a farmer's market, take time to nourish your body and find balance in this fast-paced world that we live in. Read on to discover how you can make a difference in your own health.

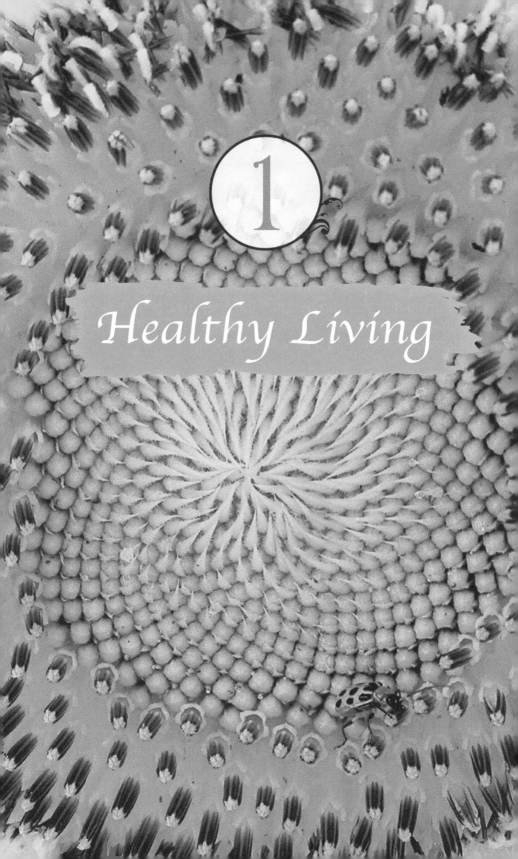

1

Healthy Living

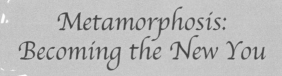

Metamorphosis: Becoming the New You

Have you made New Year's Resolutions only to find within a few weeks old habits have crept up again? Making positive changes at any time of the year takes the right mindset, determination and belief in yourself that you can do it.

Changes happen in stages. Keep your eye on your goals, dream big and you can become the New You. Nature provides a great metaphor as we look at the process of a monarch caterpillar turning into a beautiful butterfly.

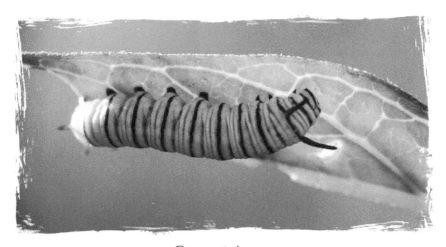

Stage 1: Instar

A young caterpillar eats and begins to grow. As it gets bigger and outgrows its form, it molts its skin five times during a process called instar.

The first step to achieving your goals is your choice. Choose to make your life better than it is today. Look ahead with the desire for change. To set your goals clearly, write them down and allow yourself to dream bigger than what you think you can achieve.

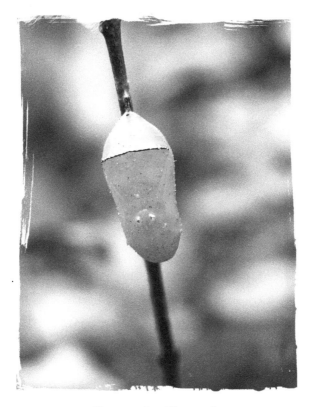

Stage 2: Chrysalis

The caterpillar has outgrown its environment and way of being and it is going through a metamorphosis. The mature caterpillar fixes itself to a safe place, hangs upside down by a tiny thread and wraps itself into a chrysalis. What exists inside the chrysalis is no longer a caterpillar and is not yet transformed into a butterfly.

How many times have you taken steps toward change and tried to bring your old way of life with you? Letting go can be so difficult but it is also incredibly freeing. What thought patterns, emotional reactions, material belongings or relationships have you already outgrown, but are still dragging around? Your old baggage will not fit with you inside the chrysalis as you go through your transformation. Sometimes what seems like an ending is really just the beginning of something greater.

To completely go through a personal metamorphosis, it is important to go inward and reflect. Get to know yourself as you unplug from the ideas of the world around you. Meditation, long baths and quiet walks in nature can aid your process of exploring your inner world.

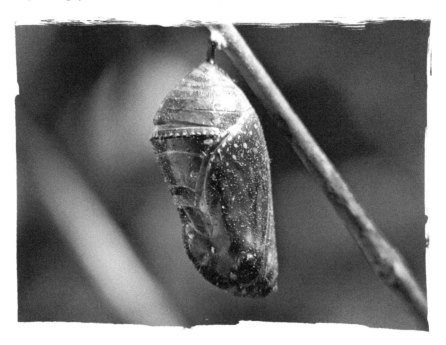

Inside the chrysalis there is quite a beautiful transformation happening. As the monarch continues to develop, the wings darken and the chrysalis becomes more transparent. Just before the monarch butterfly emerges, the entire chrysalis looks reddish black and the outline of the wings becomes more visible.

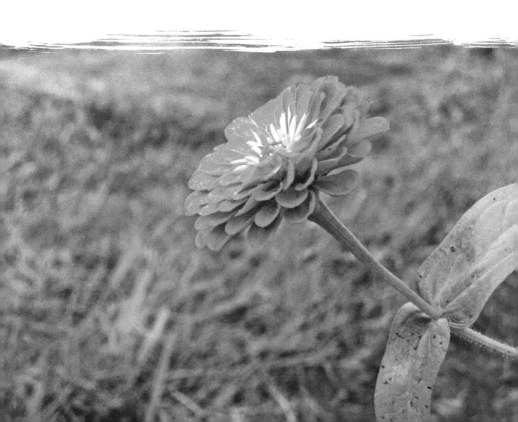

Take plenty of time in this stage to really get to know yourself, where you are going and what your newfound resolution means to you. The time of introspection before you emerge as the new you is important and shouldn't be overlooked. This quiet, reflective time is when you can gather strength to face the world and develop the stamina to stand strong in the face of resistance. Make up your mind to believe in yourself despite what the world reflects back to you.

One way to firmly set your intention is to visualize yourself having already achieved your goal. For example, if your goal is to lose weight and feel comfortable wearing a tank top in public, envision yourself in your tank top receiving a compliment from someone about how good you look. The more clearly you can see yourself in your outcome the more likely it will happen exactly the way you imagine it. Be specific, identify colors, sounds, smells and people around you and especially how you feel once you receive that compliment and really take it in.

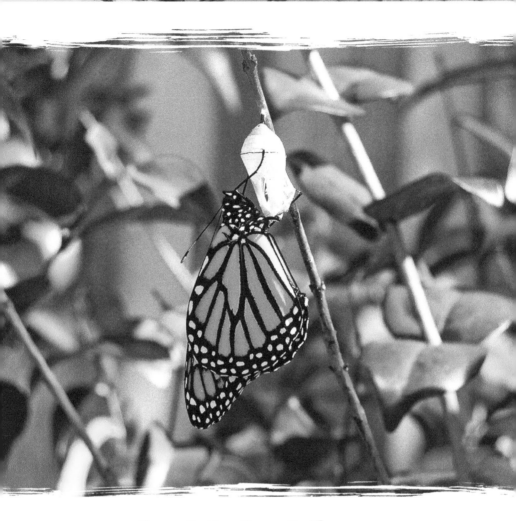

Stage 3: New Butterfly Emerges

When the new butterfly comes out it unfolds its wings and clings to the chrysalis. It pumps its wings and then attempts to fly. At first the butterfly has multiple crash landings as it navigates even the slightest wind.

How many times have you made big decisions in your life such as moving, quitting your job, breaking up with your partner, going on a diet or going back to school? As you announce your newfound path you are met with turbulence and opposition as people challenge you because they want you to stay the same—they are used to the "old you." Has this ever happened to you? It certainly has happened to me.

As the butterfly finally takes flight, it shares its beauty with the world. It pollinates our flowers and brings joy to our time spent in nature.

As you start to realize what you want to accomplish, use your imagination to dream bigger than what you think is possible. One of the simplest ways to manifest your goals is to start living your life as if you already have achieved them.

Believe in yourself. You have just as much right to be successful, happy, healthy and beautiful as anyone else. After all, if a caterpillar with stripes, legs and no wings can transform itself into a butterfly with spots and take flight, anything is possible.

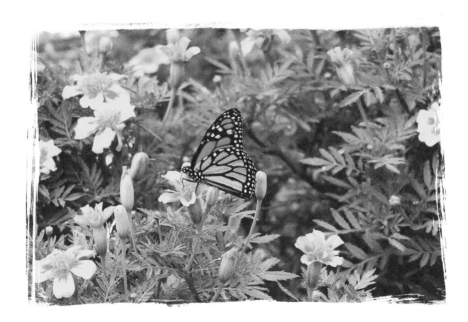

Keep Your Family Healthy with Acupuncture

Visiting an acupuncturist for the first time is an experience somewhat different from what you may be used to with other healthcare providers. Your condition will be looked at as an integrated aspect of your health, rather than an isolated symptom, which is so common in the Western medical view of the human body.

Acupuncture can be used to help hundreds of bodily conditions. Often several seemingly unrelated symptoms are addressed within one session. Each of your symptoms is linked to other aspects of your lifestyle and health. This holistic method works with your body as a whole.

Getting to the Point

All aspects of your body are connected by a system of invisible meridian lines. These are energy pathways that traverse your entire body from head to toe. Think of these like the longitude and latitude lines on the Earth. Even though we cannot see these lines, they are used to chart locations and identify geographic positions. Acupuncture meridians and points are similar.

There are twenty meridians with almost four hundred acupuncture point locations. These points mark places where the energy converges. Blocked energy can cause noticeable pain, illness, hormone imbalances, sinus congestion, depression and headaches. Health can be restored by balancing the flow of *Qi* (energy) along the meridians.

Benefits of Acupuncture

Benefit #1
Pain Relief and Improved Sleep

One of the most common reasons people come for acupuncture is pain relief. Acupuncture is a highly effective treatment that can provide rapid results for relieving pain.

After a session, it is common for people to come back and tell me how much better they are sleeping after acupuncture—even though this wasn't a specific complaint.

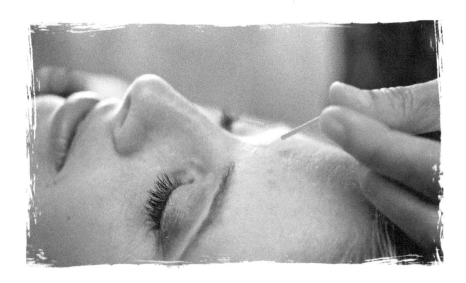

Testimonial

"Acupuncture helps so many things, but right now it is helping me recover from pneumonia & bronchitis. My lungs are loving it! I'm breathing so much better! Thank you Samadhi!"

—N.H. Cape Canaveral, FL

Benefit #2
Weight Loss

In addition to proper nutrition and exercise, acupuncture treatments can help with portion control and reduce cravings for sweets, bread, pasta, salt, carbohydrates and crunchy foods. Clients often tell me they just feel full after these weight loss treatments, and they have little desire to eat, making it easier to stick to a diet plan. This can also help when making changes in your food consumption, such as going gluten-free or switching to a raw food, vegan or vegetarian diet.

Benefit #3
Increased Energy

Receiving an acupuncture treatment for increased energy is a completely different experience than the energy boost you receive from drinking a cup of coffee. Acupuncture balances the body from the inside instead of providing an external stimulus such as caffeine. The energy lift from an acupuncture session can be helpful when quitting caffeine, nicotine or other drugs. You may notice that you have more energy during the typical afternoon slump or that you are more motivated to workout.

Benefit #4
Reduced Stress

Acupuncture treatments have a tendency to induce relaxation. One of my teachers, Chongkol Settakorn, with whom I studied in Thailand, always said that relaxation is the key to healing. The deep peace that can be attained through acupuncture sessions provides a calming response that facilitates changes physically and emotionally.

I have seen clients come in to my office for help with asthma and anxiety. Sometimes, one 30-minute acupuncture session can provide instant relief and transformation of the symptoms. It is an amazing process to witness. Clients with rheumatoid arthritis have come in with severe pain in their joints. After receiving acupuncture they can move their hands with little or no pain. Acupuncture can help with fertility, recovery from addictions, smoking cessation and many other conditions. Almost everyone reports sleeping better and feeling deeply relaxed after treatment.

Acupuncture is a natural therapy for the whole family. It is different than Western medical treatments because it helps restore balance to the entire body. From head to toe, acupuncture can be used to help people of all ages. Consider acupuncture as a natural alternative; you may be surprised at how much better you feel.

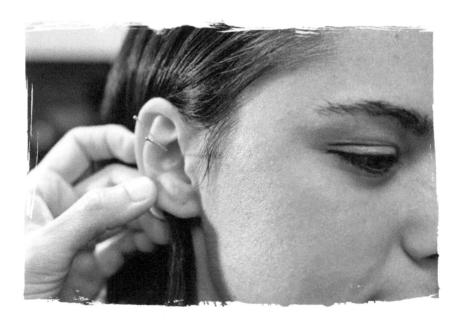

Nutrition and Iridology: Your Eyes Are the Windows to Your Health

When you see the word "healthy" what comes to your mind: feeling young again, eating the latest super foods, looking beautiful, getting out of pain, losing weight?

According to my definition, being healthy is much more than looking good and the absence of physical ailments. It is a daily practice. Every day you have a choice to give up on your exercise routine or get back to it, to eat fast food instead of fresh food, to nurture yourself or not. Your genetics, the foods you eat and your lifestyle choices are key pieces that determine your health.

By the time a symptom manifests, it is often the external sign of a long-term nutritional imbalance. When a rash, aching joints, swollen ankles or a runny nose occurs, this is the time most people realize they need to be doing something better for their bodies and decide to take action.

For example, you may have the runny nose because of a food that you ate. Joint pains might be manifesting from overuse or other dietary imbalances. Just because the symptom goes away through a suppressive medication or an herbal remedy doesn't mean "health" has been achieved. Being truly healthy is about eating the right foods and having the best lifestyle for your individual needs.

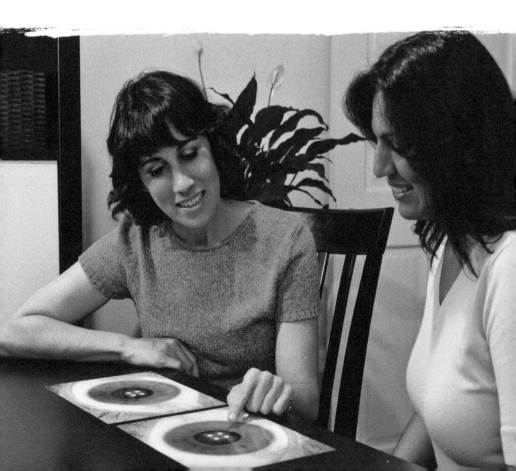

Inherited deficiencies could lead you to have digestive disturbances, issues with your thyroid gland or difficulties handling stress. It is important to support the weaker areas of your constitution to maintain the overall health of your entire body.

To experience wellness you need the right building blocks and the right lifestyle. One way of identifying the right nutritional elements for you is through a genetic assessment of the color and patterns of your eyes called Iridology.

Through an Iridology session, genetic tendencies can be identified and addressed. The signs and marking in your eyes provide insight into your DNA and can serve as a guide to which foods and daily habits are good for you as an individual. Your nutritional needs can be understood through the iris, the colored part of your eyes.

We are all born with physical weaknesses and strengths. There are dominant and recessive traits, which may or may not correlate to physical symptoms. You may have been born with a liver deficiency causing you to be very sensitive to perfumes and chemicals. Your mother may not have the same sensitivity, but your grandmother may have had liver troubles.

Sometimes a trait for a sluggish organ has been handed down but doesn't show as a physical problem. Sometimes, this will show in your eyes and can be understood by a trained Iridologist. Using iridology and Oriental medical principles, I customize food and lifestyle plans for individuals and families.

By closely examining more than one hundred areas of your health with Iridology, you can learn about the body in a unique way. Your left eye has different patterns and markings than your right eye. Each of us is truly an individual. Even identical twins have differences in the patterns in their eyes. Because you are unique, you have specific nutritional needs.

Wellness is more than the absence of symptoms or absence of disease. Health is something you build one meal at a time, one day at a time and one choice at a time. Check your Iridology health to identify exactly which foods are best for your constitution and keep you on the right path to wellness in your future.

Testimonial

"I just had an appointment with Samadhi and she was right on the money with Iridology. I was so impressed with the things that she told me. She gave me great information and insight to my diet and exercise. I have begun to implement the things that she suggested, and last night for the first time in decades, I slept for 4 hours. She is truly amazing."

—R.M., Apopka, Florida

"I made an appointment with Samadhi after I saw the report on Iridology on the Dr. Oz show. At first I wasn't sure what to expect but I was pleasantly surprised by how knowledgeable and thorough she was. She answered all of my questions and even told me about health issues I needed to be aware of in the future. I would highly recommend Samadhi to anyone wanting to become more informed about their personal health. Thanks!"

—C.L., Lake Mary, Florida

Fit into Your Skinny Jeans and Never Overeat Again

You know you've done it. You've planned to lose weight and just a few weeks later, your skinny jeans are still in the back of your closet in the *Someday, Wishful-Thinking Pile*. Maybe you have given in to late night snacking, mindless nibbling and selective memory about that candy bar you had in the afternoon. Here are some tips to help you persevere with your weight loss goals and keep you focused on looking good in those skinny jeans.

Setting your intention on a continual basis will make it easier to control meal portion sizes. Rather than a large utensil, use a small spoon or fork. Take only small bites each time. Slow down while you are eating by putting your utensil down in between bites. This will allow more time to check in with yourself to see if you are still hungry. This takes quite a bit of staying power, but it will actually build patience and discipline. Think of it as a practice in self-control. Rather than gobbling your food in a few large bites and still feeling hungry afterward, you can cultivate a deeper experience while eating and really savor and appreciate each bite.

Serve your food in the same bowl or plate for each meal. Consider purchasing a beautiful bowl, plate and glass to use for your dining experience. This will help make your meal more of a ritual than something to rush through. Start taking smaller portions of food. Wait at least 15 minutes before taking a second portion of food. Your hunger will decrease as the food digests.

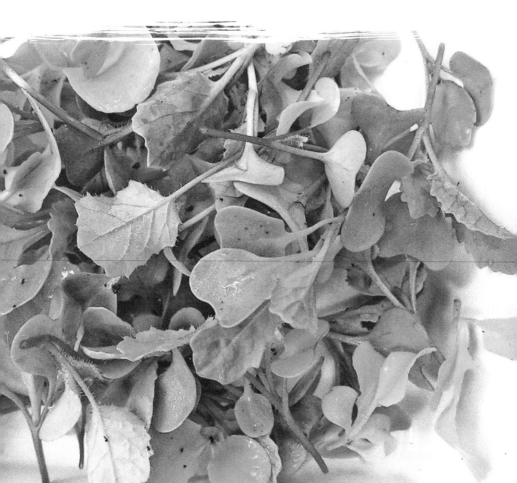

Eat in a peaceful environment with your focus on digestion. Eat at only one place in your home: the kitchen table. Do not snack while standing, watching television or any other activity. Make the focus of your mealtime chewing, consuming and enjoying your food.

Did your mother used to tell you to chew your food at least fifty times? She was absolutely right. Chew all of your food thoroughly into a paste-like consistency prior to swallowing. Allow 20-30 minutes to eat your meals, even your snacks.

Many clients tell me that they eat salad because they think it's healthy, but salads in restaurants can have high calorie counts. By the time the cheese, meat, candied pecans and dried fruits are all piled on top of that bed of lettuce with low fat dressing, you have just ordered a huge amount of calories. I do recommend eating salads, just keep them simple and don't pile on the extra ingredients.

Prepare your own food. Making your own meals is a great lifestyle practice that will help keep you on track with your goals. When you control what goes into your meal you also control what goes into your mouth. Keep healthy snacks that you like in your kitchen and get rid of the junk food. Stay out of your kitchen, cupboards, refrigerator and pantry unless you are preparing food, cleaning or putting away groceries.

Do not eat while you are driving. One client I worked with ate all of her meals on the go. From this alone, I am sure you can assume that it was all fast food that was junk food in disguise. Not only did she get all of her meals this way, but she only ate while she was driving to or from work. This is a guaranteed way to lose focus on your driving, your weight loss goals and your relationship with the food you are eating.

Avoid temptation at parties and birthdays. Instead of cake, cookies and pastries encourage your office mates to bring in fresh seasonal fruits for a treat. Although giving in to sweet indulgences may taste good, the aftereffect of the guilt isn't worth the few minutes of bliss while the flavors pass over your taste buds.

Watch out for liquid calories. Alcoholic beverages and sugary sodas are loaded with calories that won't fill you up. Eat plenty of vegetables for low calorie snacks. Allow yourself to have a small indulgence once weekly without guilt or self-judgment.

Ask your family and friends to support you. If you blow it, don't wallow in it. Go right back to your plan. Keep a good self-image and positive attitude toward life. Loving yourself will go a long way. Weigh yourself only once per week and get regular exercise. Realize that it is ultimately up to you. Invest in yourself and you will get compliments in your skinny jeans!

Uncover the Secrets to Achieving Your Ideal Weight

My clients tell me, "I start my day with coffee, skip breakfast and I am not hungry until lunchtime. I have a salad for lunch. I have another cup of coffee in the afternoon because I feel tired. I eat a large dinner with my family or friends often followed by an evening snack or dessert and then go to sleep a few hours later." Does this sound similar to how your day goes? If so, it is time for some new habits.

I will let you in on three secrets to success which I have used with my clients. The good news is this is not a diet. You won't be counting calories or weighing your food.

Secret #1
Eat a Big Breakfast and a Small Dinner

Start your day with a large breakfast. Have a snack around 10 a.m. and then eat lunch around noon. Breakfast and lunch should be your largest meals of the day. Consume the bulk of your food prior to 2 p.m. This is when you are most active and you have the best chance at burning the calories you are eating. A snack around 3 p.m. is helpful when most people experience a dip in their energy. Have a small dinner before 7 p.m. with no food afterward.

Secret #2
Eat Whole Grains

All whole grains take about 1 hour to cook. They have a hard outer coating, which is where the fiber, minerals, vitamins, bran and germ are stored. The inside of the grain is mostly starch with very little nutritional value.

My clients tell me they eat whole wheat pasta. The package says "made from whole grains" and I am frequently asked, "Isn't that a whole grain?" The answer is simply, "No." Products such as pasta, breads, boxed cereals, crackers, cookies, pastries, cakes and muffins are made from this starchy flour which provides empty calories with minimal health benefits for you.

Whole grains: rice and millet

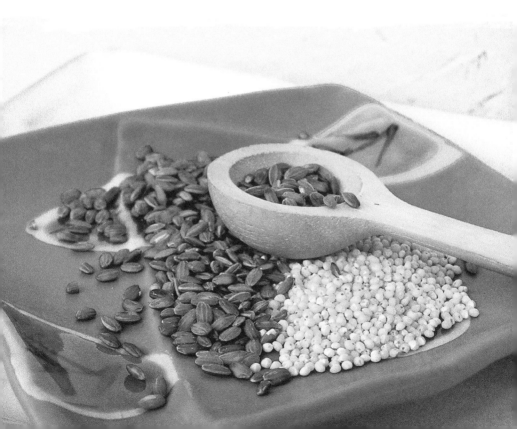

When whole grains are processed into flour, the bran and germ are ground off and separated from the remaining flour. This processing does decrease the cooking time which makes it convenient for consumers. Wheat bran, oat bran, wheat germ and oat germ are commonly sold as nutritional supplements that we pay extra money for at the health food store. Doesn't it make more dollars and sense to just eat whole grains in the first place?

The aisles in our grocery stores are lined with hundreds of non-perishable cookies, crackers, cereals and breads that are not nutritious. We have many choices of instant oats which take less than 1 minute to cook and different types of instant rice which take less than 5 minutes to cook. Processed grains contain mostly carbohydrates; they are equivalent to a packet of sugar in terms of how your body will metabolize them. I am sure if you have been around dieting and weight loss for a while you know that meals high in carbohydrates can lead to weight gain. To attain your ideal weight stay away from processed grains.

Secret #3
Go Gluten-Free

When you were younger did you ever use white flour and water to make glue? I did this in grade school for a paper maché project. Now think for a minute about what I just said: white flour + water = glue. This is exactly what white flour (which is made from wheat) does inside your digestive tract. It acts like glue. Gluten is a sticky protein found in most grains. It tricks receptors in your body to want more and more. This can lead to weight gain around your waist and difficulties losing weight.

There are only four grains that don't contain this sticky stuff. They are buckwheat, millet, rice and quinoa. These are naturally gluten-free and they won't stick to your insides or your waistline. For gluten-free breakfast ideas see the Green Smoothie recipes and Gluten-Free Hot Cereal recipe located in Section 5.

By simply eliminating gluten and substituting whole, gluten-free grains such as millet, rice, quinoa and buckwheat, you could shed unwanted pounds without making much of a change in your diet. My clients have reported losing weight just from making the switch from foods such as oatmeal to a bowl of gluten-free quinoa cereal.

Think ahead; create a menu including snacks that you can take with you. Consider cooking on the weekends and freezing portions of food you can eat throughout the week. Make a plan, stick to it and be proud of your body.

Testimonial

"I've already lost 9 pounds. I have been more conscious about eating when I first wake up and eating less in the evening and before 7 p.m. I also gave up my morning cappuccino and have been eating less in general. Hearing Samadhi speak about nutrition inspires me. She has a way of presenting the information that just makes me want to follow her advice . . . thankfully she's not a used car salesman!"

—S.V., Rockledge, Florida

Stop Counting Sheep and Get the Beauty Rest You Need Naturally

Do you occasionally feel stressed with your ongoing responsibilities and commitments to other people? Do you ever wish there were just a few more hours in each day? Does your mind race into overdrive when you finally lie down in bed each night? Although many stores and fast food places are now open 24 hours a day, you don't have to be. A good night's sleep shouldn't be classified as a luxury—it is a necessity for your good health and well being.

Getting an Early Start

Eat dinner two or three hours before bedtime. This can help with weight loss and also allows ample time to digest your food so you have an empty stomach by the time you lie in bed. This may prevent acid reflux and other digestive disturbances that could interfere with your sleep. In addition, your liver goes through a detoxification cycle in the early hours of the morning. If you are still digesting while you sleep, your liver won't detoxify effectively, causing you to feel sluggish and groggy in the morning. Sleeping with an empty stomach can improve your health and your mood.

An evening ritual will prepare your environment, your body and your mind so you can get the beauty rest you need. Make your bedroom into a sleep sanctuary and set the mood for peaceful rest. Your body produces two stress hormones, serotonin and cortisol, in response to light. Over-production of these hormones from excess light exposure can lead to weight gain around the midsection.

The ideal sleep environment is dark like a cave. Night-lights, digital clocks and cell phones with a charging light should be moved or covered. Use light-blocking curtains over your windows and just for fun consider adding a bottle of soap bubbles next to your bed to be used later on.

Now that your environment is arranged it is time for you to relax and get yourself ready to turn in for the evening.

Preparing Sleeping Beauty— Clear Your Mind

When you unwind and finish up all of your activities for the day, consider shutting off your phone, tablet and computer just after dinner and writing a to-do list for the next day. Pick out your clothing, plan your meals and errands for the upcoming day.

Winding Down with Catnip

Get into some comfortable sleepwear. Put on relaxing music and dim the lights. As part of your evening ritual, sip a cup of catnip tea. You might be thinking, *catnip*? Like I give to my cat? Yes, it is the same herb but don't go brewing up your cat's favorite toy. You can buy tea bags at your local health food store instead.

Catnip will help you unwind, reduce tension and get to sleep easier. It has a bitter taste so I suggest brewing it for just one minute and adding a touch of honey.

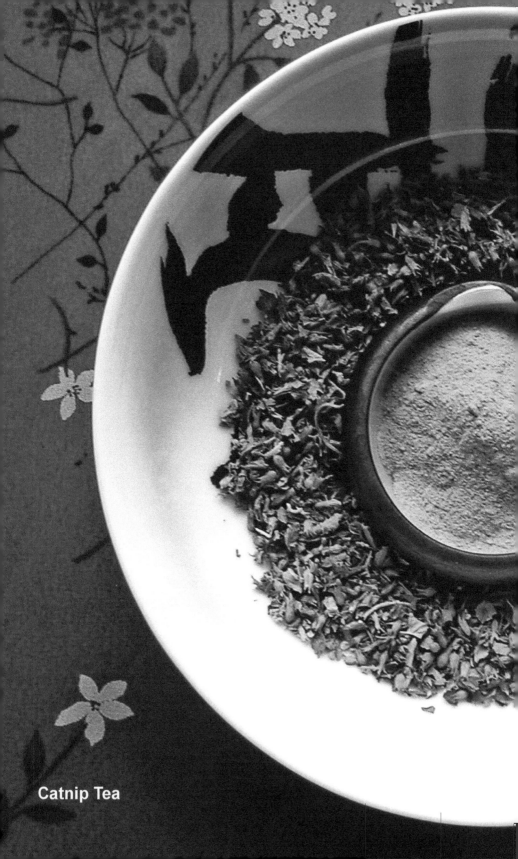

Catnip Tea

Preparing Your Body

Take time to stretch out on your bed and loosen up tightness in your shoulders, lower back and neck with gentle twisting and deep breathing. Open and close your jaw, tighten and relax your leg and arm muscles, let go of your day and your stress.

You Are Getting Sleepy . . . Very Sleepy . . .

The ancient secret to calming the mind is hidden inside your ears. There is an acupuncture point called *Shen Men* on the upper one-third of your ear. Using acupressure on this point can help you relax and quiet your thoughts. Press this point between your thumb and index finger while taking ten deep breaths. Complete acupuncture sessions can be extremely beneficial to help overcome restlessness, reduce stress and get you into a deeper sleep.

For 15 minutes before going to sleep, avoid doing anything energizing. Consider reading in bed. Choose uplifting topics such as affirmations or positive thinking. Just before you turn out the lights, open up the bottle of soap bubbles by your bedside. Take a deep breath in, and blow one bubble with a long exhale. Smile and focus on what you are grateful for. Covering your eyes with a mask or scented eye pillow can be helpful as these will draw your attention inward making it easier to fall asleep.

We are all creatures of habit. It is important to go to sleep at about the same time every night. This may be easier said than done in this fast-paced world, but start with some of these preparatory steps. Consistency will help you develop your evening beauty ritual.

Take time out for yourself in the evening. The time you invest in yourself will come back to you tenfold. You will be healthier and have more to give back to your family, work and friends. Getting a consistent good night's sleep is essential to help your body recharge, detoxify and beautify so you can be magnificent in the morning.

Testimonial

"I feel so good now...not just the headaches but everything feels better since the acupuncture session. I don't think I have felt this good in the last 5 years. I have always been tired—it is a big joke in my house that I need 16 hours of sleep a day. This is the first time I can remember that I don't feel like curling up and going to sleep. I feel amazing. I hope I keep having energy like today because it is like a second chance at life... dramatic, but that is how I feel."

—N.M., College Park, Florida

Natural Remedies for an Easy Pregnancy

Are you looking for natural solutions to help you through the physical discomforts of pregnancy? Acupuncture treatments, home remedies and self-care techniques can help you start to find relief.

Acupuncture is a safe and effective form of natural, complementary medicine that can be beneficial during all stages of pregnancy and childbirth. Compared with many Western medical therapies, there are minimal side effects and amazing benefits.

Blocked energy circulation can cause morning sickness, infertility, nausea, swollen ankles and other pregnancy-related symptoms. Acupuncture can help clear meridian pathways and restore a healthy flow of energy. This is an ancient method of accessing your body's innate healing system called *Qi*. It boosts the health of the body physically, energetically and most times, quite noticeably.

I am often asked how acupuncture works. After receiving a Master's Degree with Honors in Oriental Medicine, I can honestly say I don't know *how* it works, I just know it *does*. One of my favorite teachers in acupuncture school used to joke and say his clients would ask him, "Does acupuncture hurt?" His response was, "Nope, it doesn't hurt me one bit."

Acupuncture needles are as thin as one of the hairs on your head. Tiny sterile needles are used to affect the energy flow through meridians in the body. My technique is so gentle that most of my clients do not know I have put the needle in or taken it out.

In addition to helping you have an easier time during all three trimesters of pregnancy, one of the most valuable benefits of acupuncture is the feeling of deep peace and relaxation that can be achieved during and after a session. Many of my clients find they have the deepest rest while the needles do their "magic." Clients often state they feel like they have taken a week-long vacation during a single acupuncture session.

During the first trimester, the most common symptoms pregnant women seek relief from are morning sickness and nausea. A prenatal nutrition plan can ensure you are getting the required nutrients for you and your growing baby. Eating the right foods at the right time can help reduce the burden on your liver and calm your stomach. I recommend eating small snacks and sipping on fluids throughout the day.

One of the best remedies to soothe an upset stomach is ginger root. Fresh ginger root is available at most grocery stores. I recommend peeling it and boiling it into a delicious tea (*see recipe, page 149*).

Acupuncture is safe and effective during all three trimesters of pregnancy.

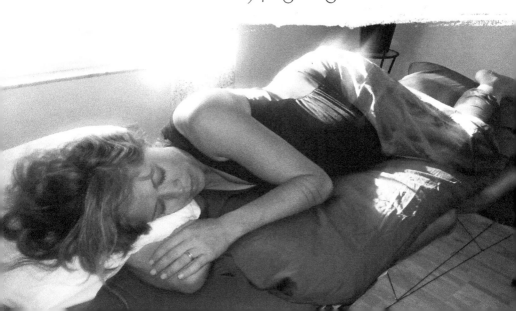

In addition to proper nutrition here is a simple acupressure method that you can do to help alleviate nausea: There is an acupressure point called Pericardium 6 located on the inside of your wrist, which can settle your digestive tract immediately. To locate this point turn your palm up. Fold your hand inward toward you to locate your wrist crease. This point is located two inches from your wrist crease inside your forearm.

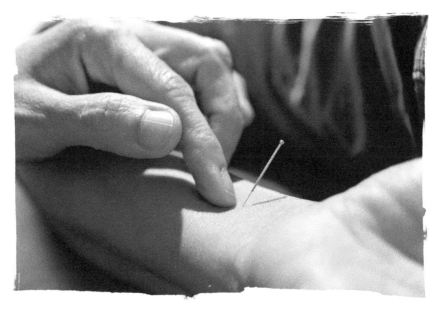

Pericardium 6: Acupuncture Point

Press this point with your thumb and hold for up to 15 minutes, depending on the severity of the nausea. Alternately, you can purchase seasickness prevention bands from any drug store. These bands are worn like bracelets around the wrists and apply constant acupressure to Pericardium 6.

Your genetics, lifestyle and nutrition will greatly influence your pregnancy. Home remedies and holistic healthcare do not replace the role of ultrasounds and regular visits to your doctors. Holistic methods are best used as supportive therapies to balance or add extra benefits to your medical care. Ginger tea, acupressure and acupuncture are safe and effective natural remedies for easing the symptoms and discomforts that arise during pregnancy.

Testimonials

"I have been going to InJoy Healthcare throughout my pregnancy for massage and acupuncture and have gotten major relief from pregnancy side effects. Samadhi has helped me with back pain, nausea, hemorrhoids, and has also given me some great nutritional advice."

—M. C., Orlando, FL

"My whole family loves Samadhi. She has been very helpful in helping us with many different types of situations. I have received great care from her during my pregnancy and when my husband's hip had been bothering him and nothing else seemed to be helping, she helped tremendously, to the point that he began playing sports that he had not played since his high school years! She is very passionate about life and her work. I highly recommend her expertise for whole body wellness."

—L.P., Lake Mary, Florida

2

Cleansing

Cleansing and Detoxification

We are all exposed to toxic substances in the course of daily activities. Common practices such as walking past a golf course that is highly sprayed with herbicides, talking on a cell phone, or experiencing emotional upset can be enough to challenge and stress the natural cleansing pathways of the body.

Fifty years ago, an image of a factory smokestack emitting big puffs of smoke was the common understanding of environmental pollution. In today's world, we are inundated with invisible toxic substances from our food, water and common household items.

With most meals, we all get exposed to pesticides, herbicides, fungicides, genetically modified organisms and radiation. Anti-microbial chemicals are commonly found on plastic kitchen items, office supplies and lining our garden hoses. Here is a list of other invisible toxic substances lurking in the average household.

- Gases from building materials
- Formaldehyde in dryer sheets
- Phthalates in body care products
- Perfluorinated chemicals in stain resistant coating on furniture
- Parabens in body care products
- Flame retardant on pillows and pajamas

While modern conveniences have made things easier for us, the detoxification pathways of the body have to deal with these invisible burdens day after day. The human body has five pathways of detoxification. They are the liver, kidneys, lymph, skin and colon. Each time you are exposed to a toxic substance it gets filtered through one or more of these organs.

Genetically, each one of us is unique. You may have inherited strong kidneys and excellent digestion but you may have a slow moving lymphatic system. You may have a sluggish colon or underactive skin. These detoxification pathways determine how your body will handle toxic substance exposure and your tendency toward ill health or good health. If the toxic burden is too great, the body will deteriorate over time.

With a healthy lifestyle, diet and proper cleansing, your body can regenerate itself well into your elder years.

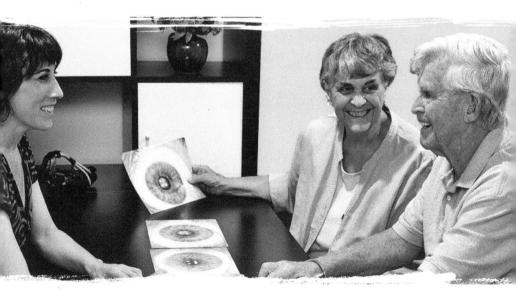

Iridology is a reliable way to learn about genetic strengths and weaknesses. By examining photographs of the eyes, the inherited ability of the body's detoxification pathways is revealed. This can be a valuable tool to determine foods and lifestyle habits that can protect and strengthen the entire body.

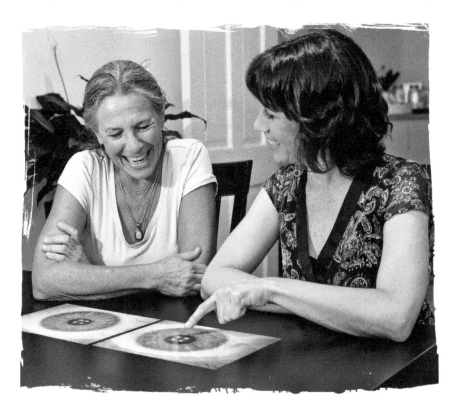

If a person was born with a deficiency in their liver and kidneys and they consume copious amounts of alcohol, the alcohol consumption will stress an already weak area of the body. This can lead to the possibility of disease to develop.

Some people have a genetic weakness in their ability to detoxify through the skin. Oftentimes, women regularly apply lotion to their entire body after a shower and then wear synthetic fabric clothing and pantyhose for eight hours a day. The skin, which is the largest detoxification organ in the body, needs to breathe. Toxins that are supposed to be eliminated through the skin can get trapped and cause deterioration in the tissues of the body. To learn more about cleansing the skin *see Body Brushing, page 40.*

If one detoxification pathway is overburdened, the others have more work to do. The skin, kidneys, liver, colon and lymph all work together and it is important to support all of them through healthy living.

Environmental toxins, chemicals in the food supply and the examples of alcohol and skin lotion represent external causes of toxic burdens to the body. There are also internal causes such as constipation, dental infections, sinus congestion, kidney stones and gallstones.

Constipation can be a serious condition that can be corrected through cleansing and proper diet. For well-being, it is essential to have healthy bowel habits and healthy eating habits. The skin, kidneys, liver and lymph provide maintenance cleansing from daily exposure to toxins. Each of these body systems eventually dumps remnants of waste into the colon where it is excreted in the stool.

Minimizing exposure to toxic substances and eating a diet of unprocessed foods are positive steps toward healthy living. It is also important to cleanse the detoxification pathways to boost the health of the entire body.

Cleansing can be as simple as drinking fresh vegetable juices for the day or as complex as methodically flushing the skin, kidneys, liver, colon and lymph over an extended period of time. The length and type of a cleanse dictates how deeply the body will purge. The feeling after a one-day vegetable juice fast is dramatically different than the feeling after a ten-day tissue and colon cleanse. Both can be effective and beneficial when done properly.

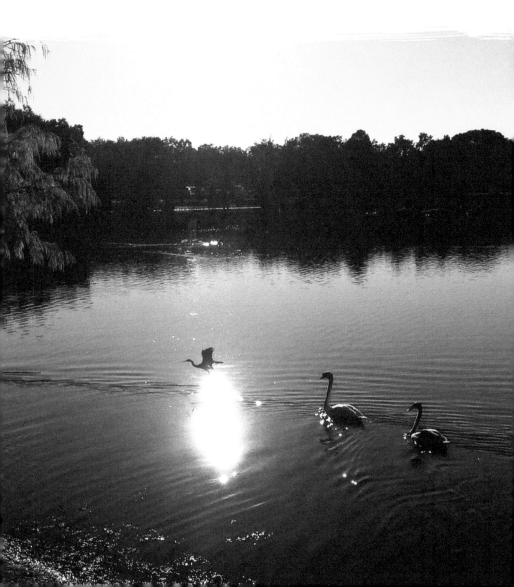

It takes time for the body to rid itself of harmful substances. The body will not cleanse without the proper circumstances and environment. Rest is essential during cleansing. The body requires time to let go emotionally, mentally and physically. Yes, cleansing the physical body does cleanse the emotions and the mind. It is possible that years of stress and debris can be washed away during a thorough detoxification program.

To get started see my suggestions for cleansing on the following pages. Each of us has a different genetic makeup and unique requirements for food, lifestyle and cleansing. If you have specific health concerns, check with a healthcare practitioner before embarking on a cleansing program.

Testimonial

"I love to read your articles. My doctor told me to do a detox and I really didn't understand what she meant until I read your article on cleansing in the Orlando Sentinel. *I just made one of the recipes today!"*

—*H.L., Kissimmee, Florida*

Silky, Smooth Skin with Body Brushing

What are your thoughts about your skin when you look in the mirror? Most of us scrutinize every blemish, brown spot, mole, patch of cellulite and wrinkle while we secretly wish for the Fountain of Youth.

I am sure you've brushed your hair many times but have you ever brushed your skin? Body brushing is one of the least expensive and easiest home remedies for softer, healthier looking skin.

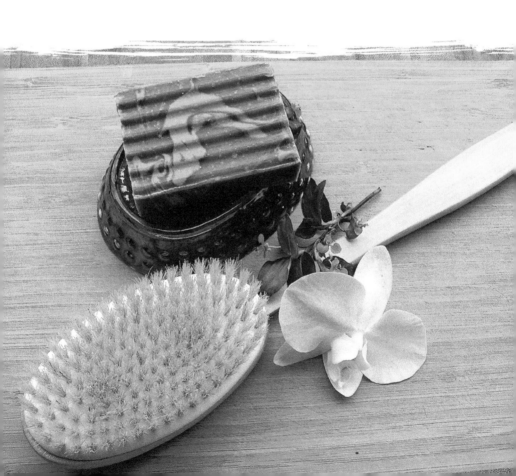

Body brushing is a beautifying and cleansing technique used to help the body eliminate toxins through the pores of the skin. Our bodies naturally detoxify over a pound of waste through the skin each day.

Body brushing is beneficial for the skin itself, as well as the lymphatic system, the urinary system and the immune system. Brushing increases circulation and therefore nutrition, detoxification and drainage throughout the body. Swollen, painful, congested or injured areas can benefit from brushing as lymph is swept away from these sites into the circulation for cleansing.

Body Brushing Basics

You will need one inexpensive piece of equipment called a body brush and these simple instructions to get started. Brushes can be purchased in health food stores and drug stores for under $20.

To find the right brush for your skin, select the brush by rubbing it on your hand to test the firmness.

Start with a soft brush and keep in mind that this is a gentle, nurturing technique.

When to Brush

Take 5 minutes to brush daily before your shower or exercise. Always brush when your skin is dry for best results.

How to Brush

Think of brushing your skin like stroking a baby or young child's skin. Gently glide your brush over your skin using straight strokes or circular strokes. Do not use firm pressure, it is better to simply repeat the strokes five times in each area. This is a gentle technique—be kind and loving to your body. Take comfort in knowing you are doing something great for your health and your relationship with yourself.

Brushing Your Extremities

Brush from your feet up toward your heart. You may prefer to sit in a chair to make it easier to reach your feet. Be sure to brush the tops and bottoms of your feet and in between all of your toes.

Brush your palms, backs of your hands and in between your fingers. Always brush towards your heart to enhance your body's natural circulation of lymph and blood.

Brushing Your Face

Use extremely light pressure when brushing across your forehead toward your temples. Brush gently down your cheeks toward your chin, and then from your chin down the front of your neck.

Brushing Your Back Side

Scrub your back up and down or however you can easily reach; a brush with a long handle will be more versatile than a shorter handle for this purpose. Brush your buttocks in a circular direction being thorough over areas of cellulite.

Take extra time to brush your joints, areas where you have scars, muscle pain, injuries and any area that can benefit from extra support. Do not brush any open cuts, irritated or sunburned skin.

Finish your body brushing session with a contrast shower. Alternate the water temperature between hot and cold for several cycles. A contrast shower opens and closes the pores of the skin; it is invigorating and rejuvenating. Finish your shower with a cool rinse.

Cleaning Your Brush

Clean your brush once a week. Fill a glass bowl with water and one tablespoon of apple cider vinegar. Immerse the brush in the cleaning solution for 30 minutes. Hang your brush outside and allow it to dry in the sun for several hours.

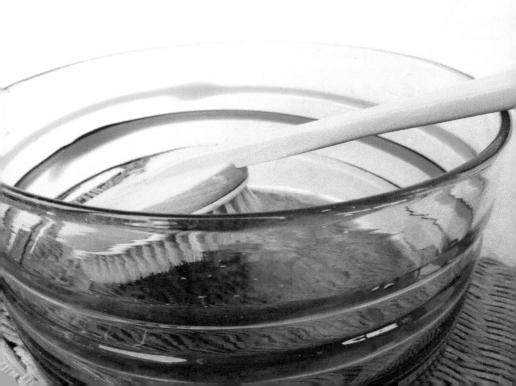

Tips for Healthier Skin in Just Five Minutes a Day

Sometimes what you do to your skin is worse than what you don't do for your skin. Most of the clients I work with tell me they slather their skin with lotion after every shower and wear tight fitting clothing for hours each day.

Let Your Skin Breathe

Topically applied oils and lotions clog the pores and don't allow the skin to breathe, sweat or detoxify. Body brushing stimulates your skin to secrete its own natural oils; you may eliminate the need for lotions and creams completely. Your skin will become silky smooth after just a few days.

Tight-fitting, synthetic fabrics such as pantyhose, spandex, workout clothes and polyester restrict circulation to your skin. Loose fitting cotton clothing will allow your skin to breathe and body brushing will encourage detoxification.

Break a sweat with gentle or vigorous exercise three or four days per week. You will detoxify through sweating and improve circulation to your skin and entire body.

Dedicate just 5 minutes each day to loving your skin through body brushing. You will love how soft your skin feels and enjoy the new glow.

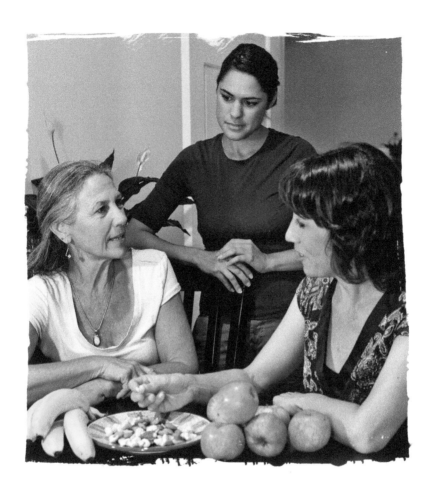

*"I thank you from the bottom of my heart for all your help. You have
helped me finally understand food and nutrition. I followed the cleanse
you designed for me and lost 10 pounds and I feel great."*

—J.R., age 87, Orlando, Florida

Super Easy Detox

Have you ever had the feeling that it was time for a cleanse? You have probably done a spring cleaning of your home, your closet and your shoe collection. How about for your body? Warm weather and the change of seasons are perfect times for detoxification. This cleanse will get rid of toxins in your body and give you a jump start to renewed health.

This Super Easy Detox can be used as a one, two, three or four day cleansing program. Follow these instructions as closely as possible. I recommend starting with the plan for Day 1 and Day 2 to boost your health. If you are interested in a longer detox simply repeat the schedule for Day 1 and Day 2 again. Longer cleanses should be supervised by a health care provider.

You may find it easiest to follow this plan on a weekend or a time when you have a few days off from major responsibilities. I highly recommend that you do not rush into a cleanse or try to squeeze it into an overly busy schedule. Shop for your ingredients beforehand and plan ahead. I cannot predict the results of your cleanse because every person responds differently based on genetics, lifestyle, health issues, medications, fitness, stress, sleep and diet. One thing I can guarantee is the more preparation, time and effort invested before a cleanse, the easier it will be to accomplish it. Take your shopping list (*see pages 50–51*) with you to the grocery and health food store. Select organic ingredients when they are available.

Quiet time, rest and extra sleep are especially important during this cleanse. The extra sleep in conjunction with the foods chosen for these recipes will help you detoxify overnight while you are sleeping. Drink a minimum of eight glasses of water throughout each day of cleansing.

My clients often tell me they are interested in cleansing but don't want to be hungry. Because so many of you have mentioned this to me, I created this program with three meals and two snacks each day. If you feel hungry, snack on celery sticks, cucumber slices or other raw vegetables to hold you over until your next meal.

Eat small portions during this program. The less you eat while cleansing, and the more you rest and relax, the deeper your body will detoxify. Eating too much food can slow down the cleansing process because your body's energy will be used for digestion rather than detoxification. This is why most of the recipes are made with blended foods. Your cleanse meals will be easy to digest since they are already liquefied.

You may find more satisfaction in chewing your blended food to enjoy the flavor of it and the experience of eating a little longer. I strongly advise against drinking from a straw because it is important to taste the flavors of your meals and snacks. Experiencing the bitter and sour flavors of these recipes on your taste buds will stimulate your body to detoxify.

The following is a suggested schedule for a two-day cleanse. I recommend getting an early start to your day. Finish dinner by 7 p.m. at the latest and get to bed around 9 p.m. Adjust the schedule as needed to suit your lifestyle. If you are taking any prescription medications, check with your physician prior to embarking on this or any other cleansing program. If you have food sensitivities or food allergies to any of the suggested ingredients omit them from the recipe. If you are interested in a specific cleanse to meet your individual needs, I can create a customized cleanse for you. Cleansing is a wise investment in your health that will pay off for years to come.

Detox Day 1 Schedule

7:30 A.M. Dry body brush for 5–10 minutes
(*see instructions, page 38*)

8:00 A.M. *Green Smoothie #1 (see recipe pages 52, 143)*

9:00 A.M. Gentle or vigorous exercise, break a sweat and
then shower

10:00 A.M. *Spicy Lemonade (see recipe pages 52, 142)*

12:00 P.M. *Savory Salad (see recipe pages 53, 128)*

12:00 to 2:00 P.M. Rest

2:00 P.M. *Spicy Lemonade (see recipe pages 52, 142)*

2:00 to 5:00 P.M. Rest, quiet time, relax

5:00 P.M. *Tomato Soup (see recipe pages 53, 132)*

8:00 P.M. Epsom salt bath: add 2–3 cups of Epsom salt
to warm bath water and soak for a minimum of
15 minutes.

9:00 P.M. Bedtime

Detox Day 2 Schedule

7:30 A.M. Dry body brush for 5–10 minutes
(*see instructions, page 38*)

8:00 A.M. *Green Smoothie #2 (see recipe pages 54, 144)*

9:00 A.M. Gentle or vigorous exercise, break a sweat and
then shower

10:00 A.M. *Bittersweet Green Drink (see recipe
pages 54, 147)*

12:00 P.M. *Blood Builder Green Drink (see recipe
pages 155, 46)*

12:00 to 2:00 P.M. Rest

2:00 P.M. *Green Energy Booster (see recipe pages 55, 145)*

2:00 to 5:00 P.M. Rest, quiet time, relax

5:00 P.M. *Liver and Gallbladder Cleanser Salad
(see recipe pages 56, 129)*

8:00 P.M. Epsom salt bath: add 2-3 cups of Epsom salt
to warm bath water and soak for a minimum of
15 minutes.

9:00 P.M. Bedtime

Detox Day 1 Shopping List

Select organically grown ingredients when available.

apple cider vinegar, raw
(2 teaspoons)

banana (1)

blueberries, fresh or
frozen (1/2 cup)

body brush

brown rice syrup or raw
honey (1 teaspoon)

cayenne pepper
(1/8 teaspoon)

celery (1 bunch)

chia seeds (2 teaspoons)

cucumber (1)

epsom salt (1 package)

flax seeds (2 teaspoons)

garlic (1 bulb)

lemons (2)

lettuce (2-4 cups)

olive oil, extra virgin,
cold pressed
(6 tablespoons)

radishes (3)

scallion (1)

spinach (1 bundle)

tomatoes (3 large)

turmeric root powder
(2 teaspoons)

salt, Himalayan (pinch)

water (2 gallons)

Detox Day 2 Shopping List

apples, red (2)

bananas (2)

cherries, fresh or frozen
  (1 cup)

cherry tomatoes (5)

dandelion greens
  (4 bundles)

epsom salt (1 package)

flax seeds (2 teaspoons)

garlic (1 bulb)

lemons (2)

olive oil, cold pressed,
  extra virgin
  (3 tablespoons)

oranges (2)

parsley (4 bundles)

pumpkin seeds
  (3 tablespoons)

salt, Himalayan (pinch)

water (2 gallons)

Day 1 Recipes

Green Smoothie #1

large handful of spinach

½ cup fresh or frozen blueberries

1 ripe banana

1 teaspoon turmeric root powder

1 teaspoon flax seeds

1 teaspoon chia seeds

Put all the ingredients into your blender and cover them with water. Blend until smooth. Drink your breakfast slowly, be sure to chew before swallowing as this will aide your digestion and help you feel full.

Spicy Lemonade

juice of 1 lemon

1/8 teaspoon cayenne pepper

1 teaspoon chia seeds

1/8 teaspoon turmeric root powder

2 cups of water

1 teaspoon raw honey or brown rice syrup

Add water to a wide mouth bowl. Roll your lemon on the counter or cutting board to loosen the flesh and then slice it in half. Place a mesh strainer over the top of the bowl and squeeze the lemon over the strainer to catch the seeds. Add the rest of the ingredients to the liquid mixture, stir vigorously and drink immediately.

Savory Salad

2-4 cups baby lettuce

1 scallion, chopped

1 rib of celery, chopped

3 radishes, chopped

2 tablespoons extra virgin, cold-pressed olive oil

2 teaspoons raw apple cider vinegar

1 teaspoon ground flax seeds

½ cucumber, peeled and chopped

Place all of your prepared vegetables and toppings into a large bowl, toss and eat.

Tomato Soup

3 large tomatoes

2 tablespoons extra virgin, cold pressed olive oil

1 teaspoon chia seeds

1 tablespoon turmeric root powder

2 cloves of garlic, peeled and crushed

1 teaspoon raw honey or brown rice syrup

pinch of salt

Put all the ingredients into your blender and purée until smooth. You can have this meal raw (right from the blender) or, if you prefer, you can warm it in a saucepan on the stove.

Day 2 Recipes

Green Smoothie #2

1 banana

juice of 1 whole orange

2 cups parsley, chopped

Blend banana and orange juice together. Add parsley and liquefy for 2-4 minutes.

Bittersweet Green Drink

1 bundle of parsley, chopped

1 bundle of dandelion greens, chopped

2 red apples

1 quart water

Core apples and cut into small chunks. Add 1 quart water and apple chunks to your blender and liquefy these ingredients first. Add the chopped greens to your blended apple mixture and liquefy for 2-4 minutes.

Blood Builder Green Drink

2 cups dandelion greens, chopped

1 cup frozen cherries, pitted

1 orange, peeled and deseeded

1 small banana

water

Put cherries into your blender and let them thaw for 15 minutes. Place orange and peeled banana in the blender. Cover all the fruit with just enough water to rotate the blade of the blender when you turn it on. Blend until creamy. Add dandelion greens and liquefy until it is a smooth consistency.

Green Energy Booster

½ bundle parsley, chopped

½ bundle dandelion greens, chopped

1 tablespoon fresh garlic, chopped

2 tablespoons lemon juice

1 quart water

Place all of the chopped greens, lemon juice and water into a bowl. After soaking for 1 hour strain the solids and sip the chlorophyll-rich liquid.

Liver & Gallbladder Cleanser Salad

½ bundle of parsley, chopped

½ bundle of dandelion greens, chopped

3 tablespoons pumpkin seeds

2 teaspoons ground flax seeds

5 cherry tomatoes sliced in half

3 tablespoons extra virgin, cold pressed olive oil

lemon juice to taste

pinch of salt

Arrange the greens on your plate and top with cherry tomatoes. In a small bowl, mix the pumpkin seeds, flax seeds, olive oil, lemon and salt. Garnish the salad with this mixture.

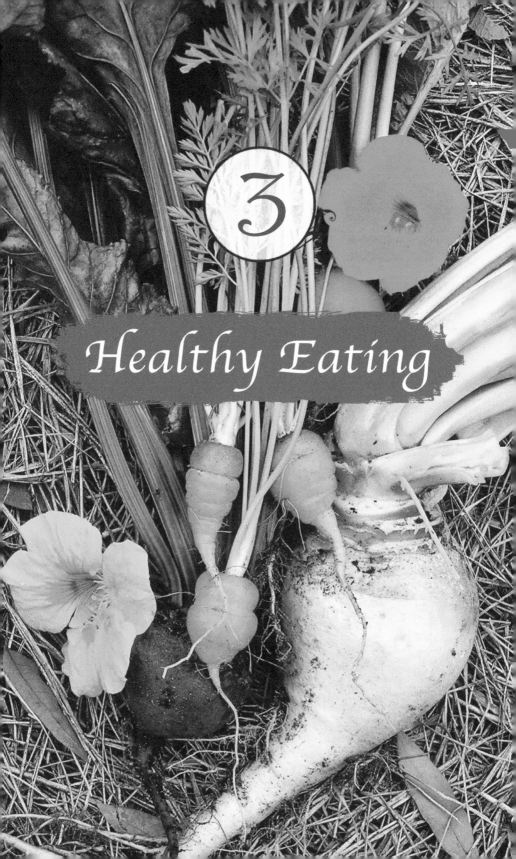

3

Healthy Eating

Eco-friendly Eating: How to Eat Healthy for You and Our Planet

Imagine walking up to a bountiful, lush garden and picking anything you want to eat. If you would have been with me any day over the last seven years, you would have enjoyed eating fresh kale, collards, cucumbers, green beans, Swiss chard and spinach right from my garden. All the stems and leaves are so juicy and plump, just bursting with nutrients! Some of the collard greens are as long as my torso—I am a petite woman, but that is gigantic in terms of vegetable measurements. Some of the leaves are almost two feet long; that gets me excited about eating lunch!

How many times have you heard the phrases, "eat foods that are in season" and "shop locally"? How do you know what is actually in season? While these trendy phrases sound like the right things to do, why should you actually apply these as lifestyle habits? Our grocery stores offer apples, bananas, lettuce, cucumbers, squash, cabbage, tomatoes, peppers and potatoes all year round, yet each of these has a distinct harvest season of only a few months within a particular region.

Every time you eat something, you have a choice. Is the food you are eating going to give something to your body or rob something from your body? Our food choices affect our individual health and the health of our Earth. Sustainable nutrition means what you eat sustains or provides for you. By my definition, sustainable nutrition also means what you are eating does minimal harm to our planet.

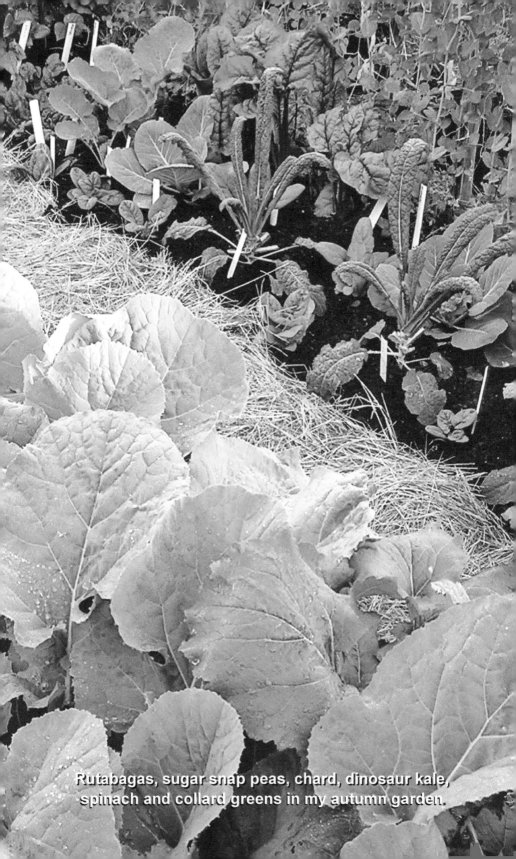
Rutabagas, sugar snap peas, chard, dinosaur kale, spinach and collard greens in my autumn garden.

There is an overwhelming amount of disposable packaging being used every single day, and for some people at every single meal. A client came in to see me and had just come from a "green" restaurant close to my office. She sat with me and ate her lunch while we chatted before her appointment. I was shocked to see for that one meal she had a plastic cup with a plastic lid for soup, a plastic plate with a plastic cover for her entrée, a plastic spoon and fork, a single serving drink in a plastic bottle, a paper bag and two napkins.

When she finished eating, she asked where the garbage can was and I said, "I will reuse those," and I did. I washed and reused all the plastic items at least one more time before their final destination in the landfill or the ocean. Manufacturers suffocate our vegetables in styrofoam packaging with plastic wrappers, much of which is non-recyclable and harmful to our ecosystems. How many times a day do you use something in a plastic, non-recyclable package and throw it away? Where is *away*? There is no *away*. Our plastic debris just gets broken down into smaller bits and ends up polluting the deepest oceans on our planet.

Sustainable Vegetables

I began teaching myself how to cook when I was in my teens. My relationship with food deepened when I became a gardener. Until I had a vegetable garden, I did not know that turnips and rutabagas had green leafy tops. Did you? They are not sold that way in stores. Many essential nutrients are in the green leafy tops that are discarded before we can purchase them.

For optimum nutrition buy root vegetables such as turnips, carrots, radishes and beets with the tops still on them. The leafy tops are completely edible, although quite bitter. All greens provide us with the dark green healing substance called chlorophyll, which is a blood purifier. The bitter flavor of leafy greens indicates they are also liver cleansers.

Do you buy your spinach and lettuce in a bag or plastic container? What do you think happens to that plastic after you eat your salad? Remember that plastic bags and containers are made from petroleum, *the same diminishing fossil fuel that is causing wars between political leaders and countries and battles over land ownership.*

Do more for yourself than cut off the top of a plastic bag, dump some lettuce on your plate, add salad dressing and call it a meal. The next time you make a salad, use some lettuce that isn't packaged in plastic. Instead of pre-washed, baby carrots sold in a plastic bag, get out your veggie peeler and get to know your produce. An even better and greener way to eat is to get to know the farmer who grew the food.

Sustainable Fruits

Most of the fruits we have access to in the stores are shipped in from other countries. They have been picked green (unripe) rather than fully maturing on the tree, bush or vine. Green fruits are still firm; they do not bruise in transport. Fruits such as bananas are picked green and then gassed. This gas causes them to ripen just in time for delivery to the grocery store, so every week when you go shopping the produce is always ready to eat. Fruits reach optimum nutrient levels, especially naturally occurring potassium, sodium and vitamin C, when they ripen completely on the trees.

Picking fruits from a local farm ensures they are in season and have been fully ripened. Often local farms have different varieties than the options that are available in supermarkets. Some varieties store well or hold up better in transport. I picked four different varieties of blueberries at a local farm, and I decided I like them all! Pick locally grown fruits in season and preserve them by freezing or canning for use throughout the year. This will provide you with the absolute best tasting fruit, which was picked at the peak of ripeness, loaded with good nutrition and will cultivate a healthy relationship with the food you are eating.

Eating perfectly ripened, fresh vegetables and fruits is the best way to get your vitamins and minerals. Many clients ask me what multivitamin I recommend. My answer is: "fresh fruits and vegetables." Eat a rainbow of colors each day. Try some different foods and learn how to prepare them.

Now imagine your next meal. There is a plate of vibrant, fresh vegetables in front of you that you've just picked from your little garden right outside your back door. You bite into a cucumber and it is so fresh and crisp that it crunches as the flavor reaches your taste buds. You don't have to worry if it has been coated with carnauba wax (as many vegetables are), you don't need to feel guilty because of the plastic shrink wrap polluting the planet, and you don't need to be concerned about how many miles that cucumber had to travel to get to your dinner plate. No, this cucumber came from your garden: the most sustainable place to get nutrition. This cucumber came from a place that provides something good for your body and for our Earth.

It is our individual responsibility to be good stewards of the Earth. Make your next meal a fresh, healthy and locally grown one and exemplify what it really means to Go Green.

Go Organic:
How to Avoid Pesticides

You know that eating more fruits and vegetables is good for you and your family. There is plenty of publicity on the antioxidants in our produce and the broad spectrum of health benefits we can get from eating fresh foods. So how do you pick the best foods for your health?

In today's world we can't judge our food on looks alone. When shopping in your local market, your instincts will likely guide you to the biggest, most perfect looking apple, pepper, cabbage or tomato. Bigger and perfect looking doesn't always mean healthy produce.

Green beans, cabbages, red winter kale and some tiny carrots from my garden

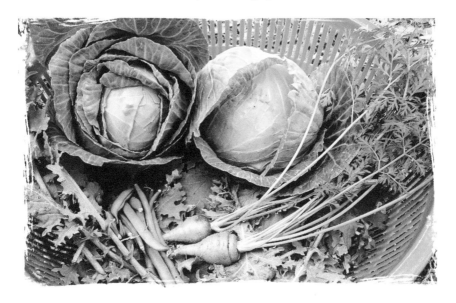

Have you ever noticed how the displays are filled with items that all look just about the same? The tomatoes are the same size with no blemishes, the pears are the same size, the orange and red bell peppers are uniformly pigmented, and all the bananas are ripening at the same rate. If you have ever seen a banana tree, you know that bananas don't all ripen at once. As a gardener, I have learned that blemishes on my produce show where the zucchini or tomato was touching the ground or a wire support cage while growing.

Have you ever wondered why the nice looking tomatoes you buy have no flavor? The reason is that they are picked green and gassed so that they don't get damaged in transport. Tomatoes from a backyard garden or local farm vary in size and shape. They are bursting with flavor and nutrients because they were ripened on the vine all the way through to maturity.

While it is nice to have beautiful tomatoes from the other side of the world in the middle of winter, the downside is we are missing out on valuable nutrients and antioxidants that the fruits develop while maturing on the plant. Buying foods that are grown locally will ensure that you are eating in-season produce with optimum nutrition.

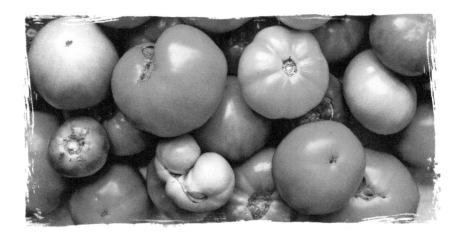

Know the Code

Upon visual inspection, organic pears look just the same as conventionally grown pears. All produce has a sequence of numbers called a PLU code found on the oval sticker or label. Codes that begin with a "9" are organic, and those with a "4" are conventional. By reading the PLU code, I have been fortunate to find organic treasures in unexpected places. I once found organic peaches tucked away in a small Spanish produce market for just over $1 per pound. It definitely pays to know how to read labels.

Vast amounts of our mass produced food is sprayed with pesticides. The Environmental Working Group (EWG) publishes a list of highly sprayed fruits and vegetables called the Dirty Dozen. The Dirty Dozen list is updated annually. Go to their website (*see Resources, page 155*) to get the most up to date information.

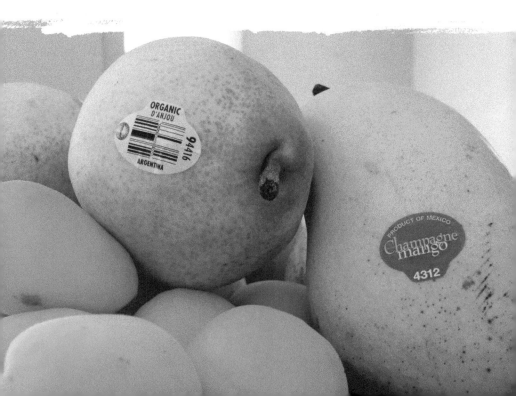

Buying USDA Certified Organic food is a great way to support organic farming. Unfortunately, not all foods that are sold commercially are being grown organically. Follow the EWG guidelines to make the best choices you can with what is available in your area.

Red winter kale, cucumbers, green beans and sugar snap peas from my spring garden

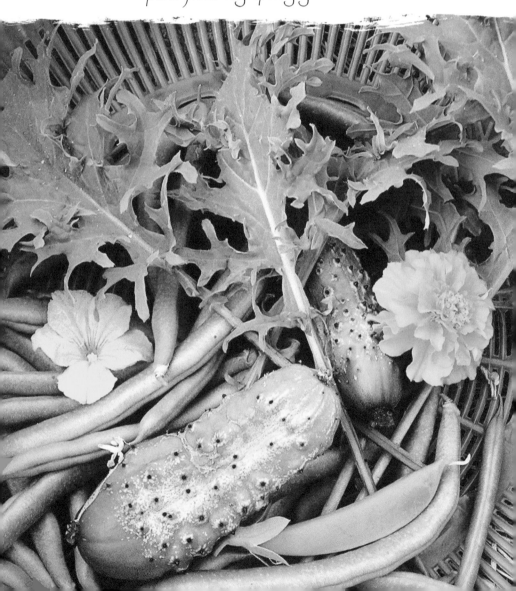

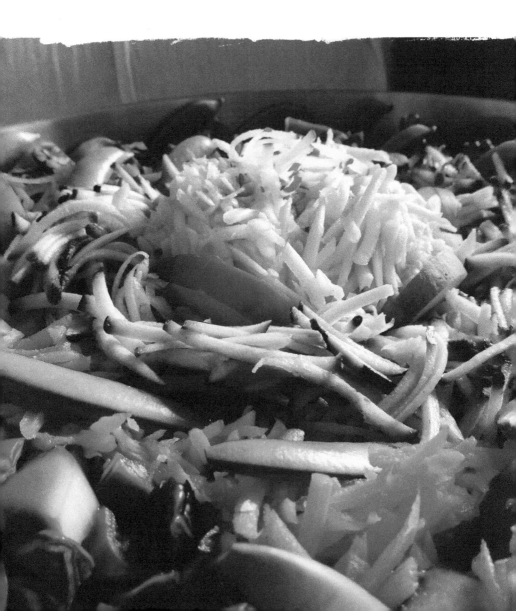

Choosing organic will ensure the safest available methods have been used to raise the food. Pesticides are not allowed in certified organic foods. Organic certification is a valuable status with a long process for farmers to obtain. There are a multitude of small farms that do not have organic certification, but use chemical-free methods to grow their food.

Check out the farms in your area and meet the people who are growing and handling your food. I love going to the local farms here in Central Florida such as Lake Meadow Naturals in Ocoee and seeing the chickens, the rows of pumpkins and then picking mulberries right from the tree.

Cabbage from my garden, very sweet and fresh tasting

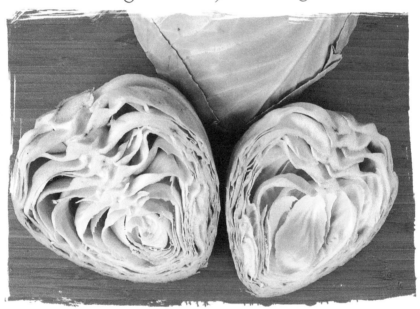

It is impossible to completely avoid chemicals in our world, but do the best you can. Buy organic, shop from local farms and try growing some of your own food. Having a garden is a great learning experience for your whole family.

Easy Steps to Becoming a Local Foodie

Your local food community is actively seeking members! A "Local Foodie" is someone who supports the local food system through gardening or buying from local markets, restaurants or farms. Here are a few easy steps to get involved:

Start a Garden and Visit a Farm

It may seem daunting to think of getting started with gardening, but one of the easiest plants to start with is the radish. You will get almost instant gratification--instant in

The first sprout of the season. Let the gardening begin!

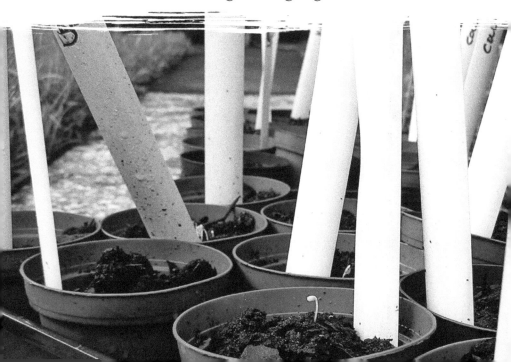

gardening terms, that is. Just one month after planting the seeds you will have beautiful radishes to add to your salads.

Seeing how other people farm or garden on their property makes it seem feasible to try it yourself. Have you ever considered growing some fresh herbs in pots on your windowsill? There are plants all around us in the surrounding landscape. Why not plant something edible?

Shop locally

There are farmer's markets just about every day of the week in Central Florida—find one in your neck of the woods. The unique quality of local shopping is that you don't always know what is available. If your local farm had an infestation of grasshoppers or too much rain, there may not be any cucumbers that week. It is this experience that can be frustrating, but it helps you feel more connected to the weather, the seasons and the community around you.

If you are used to eating tomatoes all year with no interruption, how do you ever learn that tomato plants die off when the temperature drops below 40°F? Each fruit and vegetable has a season.

Some of my favorite reasons for being a Local Foodie are:
- I have gotten to know the seasons.
- I understand my food and where it comes from.
- I feel connected to the local environment.
- I look forward to my favorite foods each season.
- I have variety in my diet.
- I am supporting the local economy.
- I know the people involved in growing my food.

Buy Locally and Eat Locally

If your friends ask you where you want to eat lunch, suggest a venue where local food is available. Many stores and restaurants are now proudly advertising locally grown food. Help grow your local food economy by building awareness that locally grown food *is* available.

At this point in time, I don't think the issue is the lack of supply or the lack of demand. Plenty of people are growing food and plenty of people are interested in buying it. This is a trend started by a grassroots effort and I am glad it is catching on in the mainstream. Ask the manager of a store or restaurant near you to start carrying local food.

So why is all this important? If you live in the United States and you buy an apple that was grown in New Zealand, think about how far that apple had to travel to get from the one continent to another, all the way to your refrigerator crisper drawer. I do, every time I eat them. Say you want to make guacamole and you found avocados from Mexico and limes from Chile. You may think you got a great deal when you purchased the limes at ten pieces for $10. But what is the true cost of those food miles?

If your food was harvested near where you live, think of the minimal resources used when compared to the transportation costs of having your food brought in from 6,000 miles away. You may not ever notice the resource costs involved in these food miles in your lifetime. We have a limited amount of fossil fuels available on our planet. When they are gone—that's it. The growing popularity of alternative energy shows the global awareness and importance of Going Green.

Every effort you make to eat locally conserves the Earth's resources. We all need to eat a variety of foods throughout the year. Do the best you can with your time and resources. Keeping your spending dollars in your local community is an investment that helps your local economy, which helps balance our global economy, our environment and the future of our population.

Picking strawberries at A Natural Farm and Education Center in Central Florida

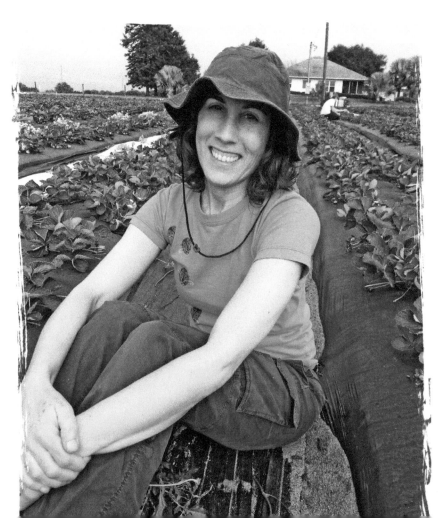

It is necessary for each of us to know the true value of healthy food. It is important to know about your spinach and understand how long it takes an avocado tree to start producing fruit. Some food can be grown in just a few months. Some trees, such as avocados, can take up to ten years to start producing a crop.

When we are used to seeing apples, strawberries and bananas in the stores all year-round, our personal relationships with these foods becomes diluted. In nature, there is a time and a season for everything.

I hope you will join the local food community in your area. Start a garden, visit a local farm and request local food at the stores and restaurants near you. Whether you believe in global warming, drive a hybrid vehicle, care about recycling or enjoy getting lettuce from your neighbor's garden, eating locally grown food is a very tangible way to Go Green.

Become a Local Foodie and support your local food economy. Take comfort in knowing you are creating a sustainable future for generations to come.

Keeping Genetically Modified Foods Off Your Plate

Genetically modified foods (also known as GMO or GM) are similar or identical in appearance to other foods we are used to seeing. They seamlessly blended into grocery stores about thirty years years ago without consumers knowing what was happening, until recently. Now this topic is out in the open and consumers are taking action by demanding GMO labeling, signing petitions and effecting change by not buying them.

The genetic modification process involves combining different types of DNA to improve crop yields, make plants more tolerant to changing weather conditions and resistant to insect invasions. There are hundreds of crops being experimented with using bacteria, viruses, antibiotics, plant, animal and insect DNA. This is cause for alarm because these are not proven to be safe for human consumption in long term studies. Although there is much experimentation, not all of these GMO science projects make it to the marketplace.

Some GM foods that have made it to the grocery store shelves have not been around for long. Years ago, the DNA from cold water fish was combined with tomato DNA, producing a GM tomato plant that was cold-hearty. This failed in the market place because consumers didn't like the flavor. Crossing a fish gene with a vegetable gene is suspect and the side effects to human health have yet to be determined.

Information on which GM foods are making it to the marketplace changes continuously. Court cases between farmers and corporations, GMO legislation and consumer demands are all shaping this issue in present time. Currently there are only a few varieties of genetically modified fruits and vegetables sold in the grocery stores. However, the bulk of the wheat, corn and soy being farmed at this point in time is genetically modified.

GM wheat, corn and soy show up in most of the boxed, processed, mass produced and packaged foods. According to the Institute for Responsible Technology, *(see Resources, page 165)*, GM ingredients are used to make things such as ketchup, vitamin supplements, veggie burgers, meat substitutes, tofu, soy milk, corn syrup, energy bars, protein powders, cereals, breads, candies, snack foods, pastries, food additives, rennet, artificial sweeteners, enzymes and more. GM grains are used as feed for livestock and poultry, which translates into meat, eggs and dairy products containing GM constituents. Buy meat, poultry and

Corn from my garden—very labor intensive to grow without chemicals, but delicious and worth every bite!

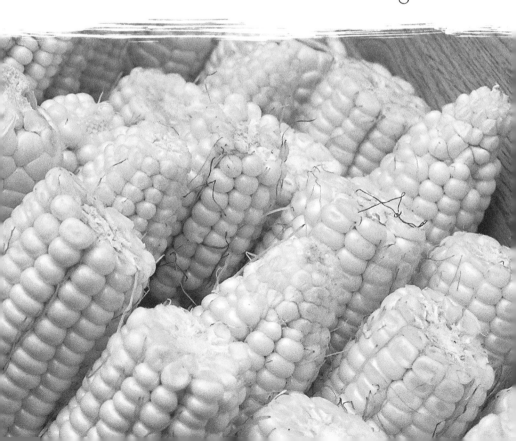

dairy from local farmers you can talk with about what they are feeding their animals so you can make an educated purchase. Farm raised fish are also fed genetically modified grains; buy wild caught fish. Other sources of genetically modified ingredients are dairy products that come from cows who have been injected with rBGH. This is a genetically modified hormone that increases the production of milk. Organic milk does not contain modified ingredients or rBGH.

I have listed resources in the back of this book if you would like to partake in GMO labeling and GMO issues that are currently being addressed. You can also get involved by buying foods that are labeled Non-GMO and USDA Certified Organic. Each of these steps makes a positive impact on the environment, the economy and your health. Remember you are voting with your dollars—make your food purchases count!

How Sweet It Is: Beginner's Guide to Carbohydrates

Do you ever wonder what type of diet to follow? There are many popular low fat diets, high protein diets and low carbohydrate diets. So how do you know which one to choose and what is best for you?

Fats, proteins and carbohydrates are the foundational building blocks of all balanced diets. Dramatically increasing or decreasing any one of these three macronutrients might help you reach a short term goal, such as weight loss or increased muscle mass. However, minimizing or eliminating carbohydrates over the long term can cause complications with kidney function and lead to a condition known as ketoacidosis. In order to maintain the health of all the body tissues, you need all three of these important food groups.

Good Carbs

Every cell in your body needs carbohydrates for energy. Many clients that see me for nutrition consultations tell me they try not to eat carbohydrates so they won't gain weight. Don't be afraid to include unprocessed carbohydrates, such as whole grains, in moderation. They provide glucose, which is the necessary fuel that your muscles and brain depend on.

Bad Carbs

Eating excessive amounts of processed carbohydrates, such as white bread and pasta, can cause imbalances in the body. It can lead to complications such as weight gain, dysglycemia (swings in blood sugar levels from high to low) or a pre-diabetic condition known as insulin resistance.

Glycemic Index

To keep your blood sugar balanced while enjoying carbohydrates, let's take a look at something called the glycemic index. Foods that have a high glycemic index have a sweet flavor, such as high fructose corn syrup. These foods will raise the blood sugar level rapidly and then once the glucose is used up, the level drops off quickly. Have you ever seen children eat candy with high fructose corn syrup in it? They get instantly hyperactive as their blood sugar spikes and then 30 minutes later, when their blood sugar drops, they get tired and cranky.

High Glycemic Index

To avoid peaks and dips in your blood sugar and your mood, stay away from foods and beverages that have a high glycemic index. Some examples of high glycemic foods are sugary sodas, bread, pastries, cookies, pasta, honey, fruit juices, cantaloupe, tropical fruits such as mango, pineapple and banana, desserts made with sugar, flaked cereals, crackers and jam. Although it doesn't taste sweet, white bread has a high glycemic index because the wheat used to make the bread is highly processed. Whole grains such as quinoa or millet have a lower glycemic index than products like crackers, pita breads, tortillas and pasta. For example, a bowl of quinoa, rice or millet has a lower glycemic index than pasta made from quinoa or crackers made from rice.

Moderate Glycemic Index

Moderate glycemic index foods are not overly sweet in flavor and have a mild effect on your blood sugar level. Consume these in moderation. Some examples are sweet-tasting vegetables such as carrots, yams, cooked squashes, sweet potatoes and beets and fruits such as oranges, figs, peaches, pears, apples, pomegranates, apricots and plums.

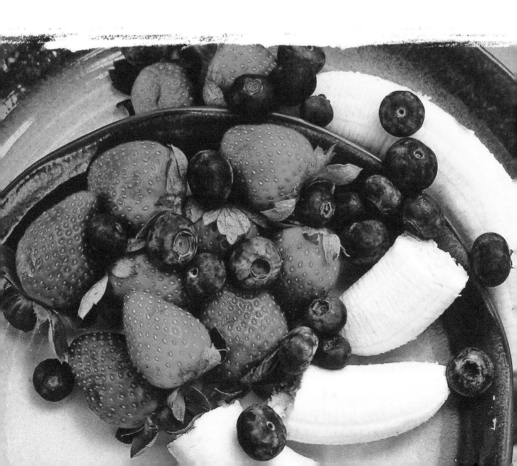

Low Glycemic Index

Low glycemic index foods cause a mild increase in your blood glucose and are much easier for your pancreas to handle. Examples of these low carbohydrate foods are: grapefruit, lemon, lime, sour cherries, strawberries, raspberries, blueberries, whole grains such as barley, quinoa, millet, legumes and vegetables such as cucumber, kale, collard greens, celery and lettuce.

Most of us like something sweet. If you must use a sweetener, try stevia as it has a zero glycemic index. Even though it has a very sweet flavor it will have no effect on your blood sugar level. Check your local health food store for stevia and do the research online for a more detailed listing of the glycemic index.

A diet comprised of whole grains, beans, fresh vegetables, fresh fruits, raw nuts and seeds provides a good blend of carbohydrates, proteins and naturally occurring, healthy fats. If you are a diabetic, please consult with your healthcare provider before making any dietary changes.

For better health, it is definitely important to be aware of the glycemic index of the foods you are eating. Get to know what you are buying. Read labels and watch out for added sugar. Words that end in "-ose" are sugars, such as high fructose corn syrup. Choose unprocessed, whole foods and keep your sugar in check.

Get the Skinny on Fats and Oils

Trans-fats, hydrogenated oils, polyunsaturated fats, fat free... when did we all need to become chemists just to understand how to read the label on a jar of peanut butter?

The labels on packaged foods are now designed to bring our attention to nutrition messages such as zero trans-fats, low cholesterol, low fat and fat free. The very fact that these products are *in* a package and *have* a label should indicate that some processing has been done and, therefore, some nutritional value has been lost. Instead of trying to be a food detective when reading labels, find foods that don't need a label. Foods that look like they did when they came out of the ground, off of a tree or bush are going to have the best nutrient content.

Chia, sunflower, flax and pumpkin seeds

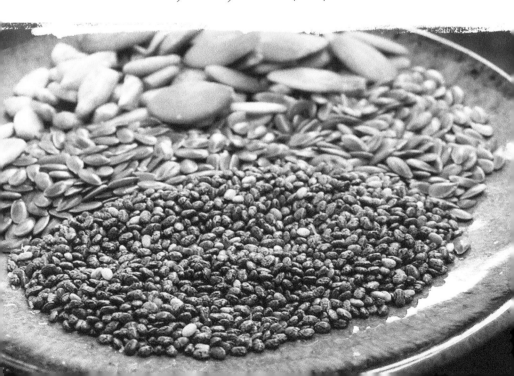

Selecting the Right Fats and Oils

There are many different types of fats and oils. At room temperature fats are solid and oils are liquid. For simplicity, I will discuss saturated and unsaturated fats. Saturated fats naturally occur in avocados, dairy products, animal proteins and nuts. The structure of saturated fats tends to be stable and stay about the same when exposed to moderate heat.

Unsaturated fats naturally occur in olives, pumpkin seeds, sunflower seeds, flax seeds and hemp seeds. The molecular structure of unsaturated fats is unstable when heated, meaning it changes even at low temperatures.

Raw vs. Roasted

When all oils and fats are heated, they reach what is called a smoke point. The temperature at which this happens varies, depending on the molecular structure. When fats and oils reach their smoke point they turn into trans-fats. Trans-fats are damaging to cell membranes of the body and are suspected to be carcinogenic.

Omega 3 essential fatty acids naturally occur in olive oil. Most people have heard this is good for them so they cook their food in it. Olive oil is a type of unsaturated oil that is unstable when heated past its smoke point of about 100°F. Most skillets get up to 750°F, which is important to keep in mind if you sauté or stir fry.

The best way to eat fats and oils is in their raw, unheated, unroasted and unadulterated state. This might sound easier than it is to apply. Even cold pressed oils get quite hot during the extraction process, often well above several hundred degrees, turning them into unhealthy trans-fats before the oil ever makes it into the bottle.

A good guideline is to keep your oils away from heat. If you are going to sauté, plan to slow cook at the lowest heat setting possible. Even better, consider steaming, baking or boiling your food to cook it at lower temperatures. Add your oil as a garnish when you are done cooking, then you will reap its health benefits.

Fats are Good Fuel

I am frequently asked, "Does eating fat make you fat?" The answer is, "In moderation, no, it doesn't." Of our three main food groups (fats, proteins and carbohydrates), fats have the most calories. The good side of this is calories provide fuel and energy. One of the benefits of eating fats and oils is long-term energy.

Raisins, walnuts and coconut

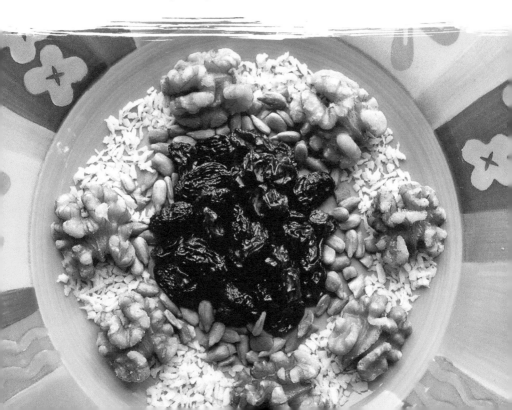

If you eat a piece of watermelon, which is a carbohydrate, your blood sugar will spike a little and then drop off in about 30 minutes. When you eat an avocado, which is a fat, there is no blood sugar spike. Because fats are higher in calories your energy will last much longer than 30 minutes, which can be helpful for long workouts or in cases of low blood sugar.

You are unique. Each of us has different nutritional needs. Not everyone should eat all types of fats and oils. For example, many clients I work with have gallstones or have had their gallbladders removed. This directly affects their ability to break down and metabolize fats and oils.

Coconut oil has a unique molecular structure. It helps regulate cholesterol and also helps burn fat for those on weight loss programs. This type of oil in particular is easy for most people to digest. For more information on the health benefits of coconut oil *see Coconuts, page 115.*

Flax oil and hemp oil are wonderful sources of anti-inflammatory Omega 3 essential fatty acids. Regular intake of these can be helpful in cases of mood disorders, depression and arthritis. If you stretch your imagination a bit when eating toast with flax oil, you might find that it resembles the flavor of melted butter. For people who are intolerant of casein, which is a protein in dairy products, this is a healthy alternative.

Nuts and seeds are a fantastic source of protein on a plant-based diet. They are complete packages of nutrients classifying them as a meal all by themselves. All nuts and seeds are high in beneficial fats, minerals and vitamins, which benefit the organs, glands and tissues of the body. They offer a high content of calcium, selenium, zinc, vitamin A and vitamin E. If you have a nut allergy, do not eat nuts.

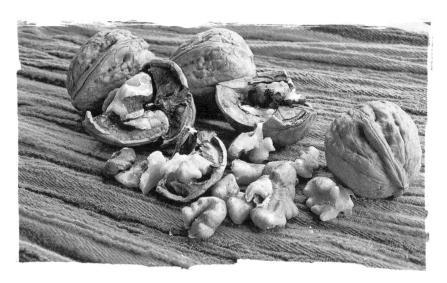

Walnuts in the shell

Tips for Eating Nuts and Seeds

Walnuts, pecans and almonds contain tannins on their outer skins, which can irritate the digestive tract. Soaking them for a few hours in water will soften the nuts, remove the tannins and make them easier to digest. Soaking also begins the germination (sprouting) process and changes the nutrient content favorably, increasing the protein content and decreasing the fat content. Almonds can also be dropped into boiling water for 1–2 minutes. When they cool, the skins with the tannins can be easily slipped off. The inner nut is softer and easier to digest.

Be sure to chew well so you get all the nutrients inside the nuts. If you don't soak your nuts and seeds, I suggest grinding them into a meal using a coffee grinder. Nut and seed meal can be enjoyed by sprinkling it onto food, such as a bowl of oatmeal, rice or a salad.

Sunflower seeds

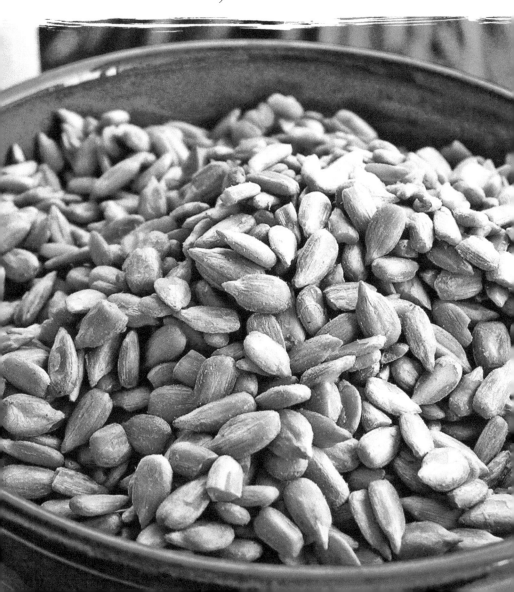

Nut and Seed Butters

Butters made from almonds, cashews, sunflower seeds and sesame seeds (tahini) are a wonderful way to enjoy the health benefits of nuts and seeds. The *Raw Halvah* recipe (*see page 138*) offers a quick and easy tahini dessert. Most nut and seed butters are roasted, not raw. Roasted nuts and seeds release a higher yield and are more flavorful. The sacrifice for this delicious flavor is in the health benefits. Fats and oils that have been heated past their smoke point are trans-fats. Find raw nut and seed butters at your local health food store.

There are health benefits to all types of fats and oils, especially when eaten in moderation. The next time you are shopping, head toward the bulk bins and produce section to get your raw nuts and avocados: no labels, no marketing messages, just good nutrition.

Testimonial

"By the time I made my appointment with Samadhi, I had already tried 4 nutritionists, 2 iridologists, 6 dermatologists and a few specialized doctors. Traditional medicine gave me a temporary bandaid for my symptoms but nothing that would help my acne long term (and more importantly, find the cause) and they were also unable to control my anxiety without affecting my personality from medication side effects. Only a few months after following Samadhi's recommendations and treatment, I was already seeing results with my skin and my anxiety. She really guided me throughout the whole process and was so helpful with my new diet and my new life. Other practitioners will overload with supplements, however, Samadhi was very reasonable and it was never too much to handle. The process was so emotional for me since I have struggled with anxiety and acne for almost 15 years. She was so understanding and it is so apparent that she really wants to help people. Almost 7 months later, I find myself with CLEAR SKIN without having to take any prescription drugs and my anxiety is getting better every day."

—M.D., Winter Park, FL

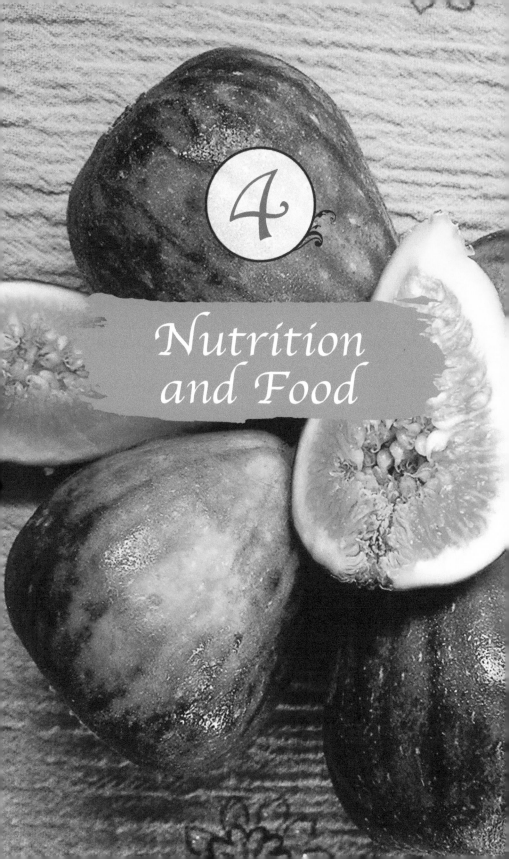

4

Nutrition and Food

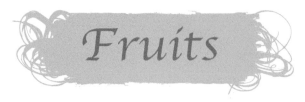

Fruits

Mango

Are you looking for a natural alternative to satisfy your sweet tooth? In Florida we have the great opportunity to enjoy tree-ripened mangoes for a few months starting in late summer. Imported mangoes are available year round. Whether your mangoes are from a local grower or or the nearest grocery store, here are a few tips for selecting and enjoying this delicious fruit.

Selecting Mangoes

Select large fruits that yield to gentle pressure. If the mangoes are still hard, keep them at room temperature to allow them to ripen. When they start to soften, you can transfer them to your refrigerator to slow the ripening process. Then you will have an extra few days to eat them.

Depending on the variety, mangoes can have different colored skin; they can be red, yellow, peach or green. Red pigment does not indicate ripeness or sweetness of a mango. My favorite varieties grown in Florida are Kent, Tommy Atkin and Hayden because they are creamy and sweet. I also find the imported Ataulfo variety to have great texture and flavor.

Some mangoes have marks on the surface, blemishes on the skin or sap oozing from the stem end. Small blemishes will not affect the flavor of the fruit, but avoid fruit with large black spots. Be careful while handling mangoes with oozing sap because it can irritate sensitive skin. Do not eat the mango skin or mango pit.

How to Cut a Mango

Divide the mango into three pieces by making two cuts along the sides of the flat, oval-shaped pit.

Make cross cuts in the flesh like you are drawing a tic-tac-toe board with your knife. Push on the back of the fruit and the sections will be easy to eat right out of the skin.

Mangoes are high in vitamins A, B and C and the trace mineral copper, which is helpful for building the blood. For me, the bottom line is that mangoes taste delicious and make a great substitute for sweets and ice cream (*see Mango Lime Sorbet recipe, page 134*).

Mangoes from Local Roots grown
in Central Florida . . . delicious!

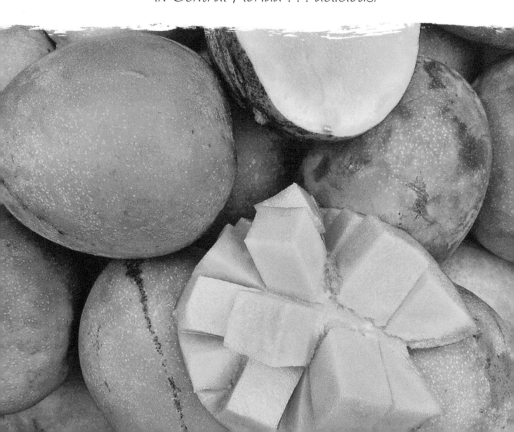

Orange

Selecting and Storing Oranges

Have you ever wondered why the oranges in the produce department are all exactly the same color? Choosing them can be a little deceiving because the color of the peel is sometimes enhanced with dye. Oranges from a local grower have a high likelihood of being fresh and unprocessed.

I am generally not concerned with blemishes, dirt or other debris visible on the outside of the fruit, especially when I have picked them myself from a neighbor's tree and know I will wash them. Try to select oranges that yield slightly when being gently squeezed.

If the oranges are firm just keep them at room temperature until they soften. When they start to yield with pressure, they can be transferred to the refrigerator for longer cold storage.

Nutritional Benefits of Oranges

When you think of a fruit that contains vitamin C, oranges and orange juice probably come to mind. Most people only want the orange-colored flesh and juice and discard all the nutritional goodies in the outer layers of the fruit. I am sure you are accustomed to eating the sweet orange sections, perhaps a little bit of the white strings and have occasionally bitten into a seed. The entire orange from seeds to peels is edible.

Orange Peels

If you are going to ingest a little bit of the peel it is essential to get unwaxed, organic oranges. Some store bought citrus is coated with carnauba wax. If you want to check for wax, simply scrape the peel with your fingernail. If it is coated, the wax will flake off.

The peel contains the essential oil limonene. In very small doses, it is an excellent liver cleanser. Recipes calling for citrus zest give you just a small amount that shines through with robust flavor, adding zing to your cake, frosting or entrée. Too much limonene can be hard on your stomach and your tooth enamel, so enjoy it sparingly.

Red navel oranges from my neighbor's tree

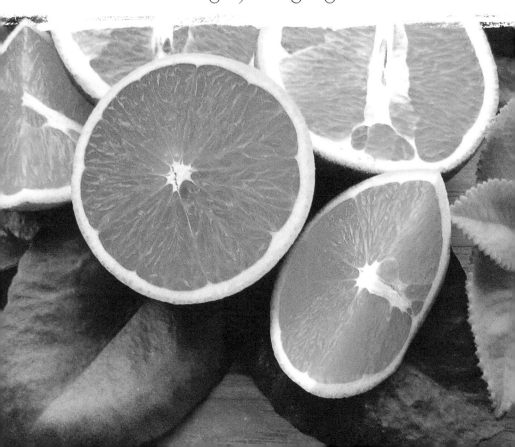

Orange Pith

Try eating a little of the white pith that comes between the fruit and the outer peel, just watch out for the intense bitter flavor. The pith contains bioflavonoids such as rutin and hesperidin, which are part of the vitamin C complex. You may be buying these as a nutrition supplement when there is great natural food source in the produce department, or, if you're lucky, from your neighbor's back yard orange tree.

Orange Seeds

Orange seeds are edible, but so much of the citrus we have access to has been hybridized. Hybridization is a process of combining two or more plants to encourage the best traits to emerge. If you are fortunate to find an orange with seeds in it, try snacking on one or two instead of discarding them. The seeds contain a small amount of protein and fat and also have quite a bitter taste, indicating liver cleansing properties.

Orange Juice

If you have the option to get your juice with the pulp in or out, I recommend the added fiber the pulp has to offer. Pulp-free juice (especially when pasteurized instead of freshly squeezed) is high in naturally occurring fruit sugars. The pulp and the other parts of the orange already mentioned will balance out the sweetness of the fruit. Orange juice makes a great addition to smoothies and salad dressings. See recipes in Section 5 for a new twist.

Persimmon

When persimmons come back in season each year it is like visiting one of my old friends. You will find two varieties of persimmons sold in stores: Fuyu and Hachiya. Acorn-shaped Hachiya persimmons have an astringent property (when they are still firm) that is unpalatable. Before they ripen, they have an unpleasant, sticky grit that adheres to the inside of your mouth.

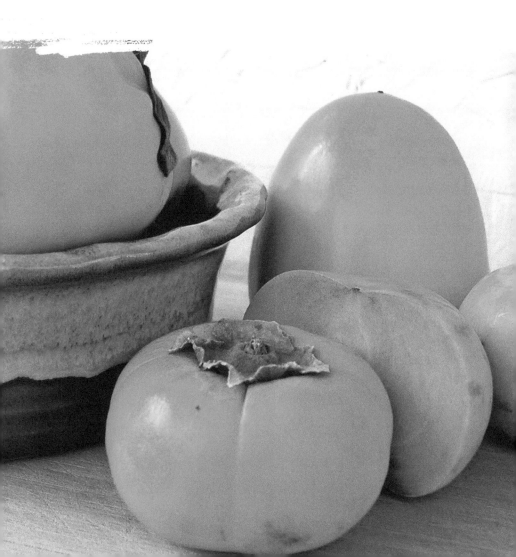

I recommend Fuyu persimmons that look like orange tomatoes. Fuyu persimmons are much sweeter than Hachiya and don't have the astringent property.

Selecting Fuyu Persimmons

Fuyu persimmons can be eaten when they are soft or hard. I buy them at all different stages of ripeness. I like to eat them over the course of several days and want them to be ripe when I am ready to eat them. When they soften they get very sweet and almost turn into a liquid gel.

Sometimes I will select the ugliest persimmons on display (those covered with brown spots and bruises) because they are ripe, ready to eat, have a great texture and sweet flavor. Firm persimmons travel well as a snack that can easily be eaten like a pear or apple.

The seeds and skins can cause digestive upset and should not be eaten.

Persimmons are high in fiber. They provide vitamin C, vitamin A and manganese, making them both nutritious and delicious to eat.

Storing Persimmons

Keep the firm fruit at room temperature until it softens. When I have stocked up on persimmons and have a big pile of fruit, I like to keep them on a plate and check them each day by turning them over and gently squeezing them to test the softness. As soon as they begin to soften I transfer them to the refrigerator to slow the ripening process until I am ready to eat them.

Preparing Persimmons

Firm persimmons can be sliced open with a small knife. I like to use a paring knife and eat the pieces much like a sliced orange, avoiding the pits and the skin. Soft persimmons will be juicy and mushy and I find it less messy to open them over a plate. This is helpful to catch the juice.

Eating Persimmons

My favorite way to eat persimmons is to peel back the skin and start chomping. If you are lucky enough to visit a u-pick persimmon farm you can stock up and freeze the extra fruit. This way you can have some to snack on during the season and some to freeze for a treat later in the year. Persimmons can be blended into an easy, delicious pudding (*see Persimmon Pudding recipe, page 135*).

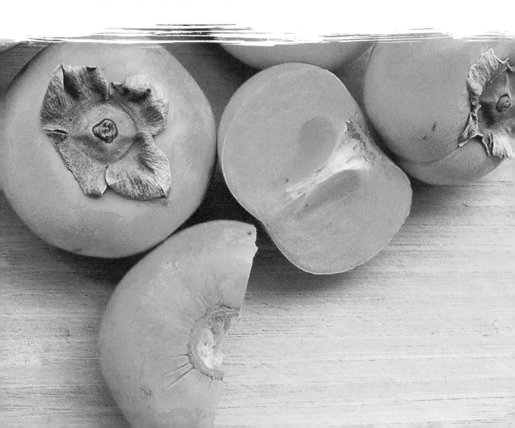

Strawberries

Do you remember when you were a little kid how everything seemed bigger? I wish you could have seen the huge strawberry fields in New York when I was growing up. I would go to the u-pick with my family for our summer ritual when the strawberries were in season. We would pick so many that the entire kitchen smelled like a strawberry paradise. In my youth, eating seasonal food was fun and exciting. As a gardener and health care provider, I have realized the importance of buying fresh food from local farms and the positive effect this has on our health, our local economy and our global ecosystem.

Selecting Strawberries

Select strawberries that are red from the tip of the fruit to the stem. Avoid moldy, damaged berries or packages leaking strawberry juice. Strawberries are fragile and they can deteriorate quickly. The following rinsing guidelines will help your berries stay free of mold and stay fresh longer.

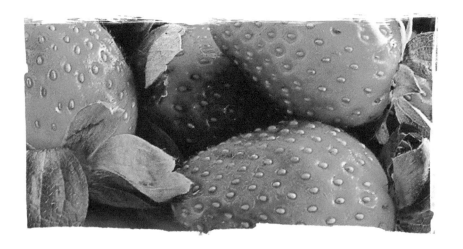

Rinsing and Storing Strawberries

Fill a large bowl with strawberries and water. Add a tablespoon of raw apple cider vinegar. Soak your berries for ten minutes and then pat them dry. Refrigerate your berries in a container with a paper towel lining the bottom. These two steps will prevent mold from growing on your berries. If you don't eat them within a few days, repeat the vinegar wash, dry them and refrigerate them again. Plan to eat or freeze the berries within a few days of picking or buying them.

Freezing Strawberries

I still love to pick strawberries and stock up when they are in season. I enjoy using frozen berries in smoothies, to top a bowl of steel cut oatmeal in the morning and just plain old strawberries in a bowl.

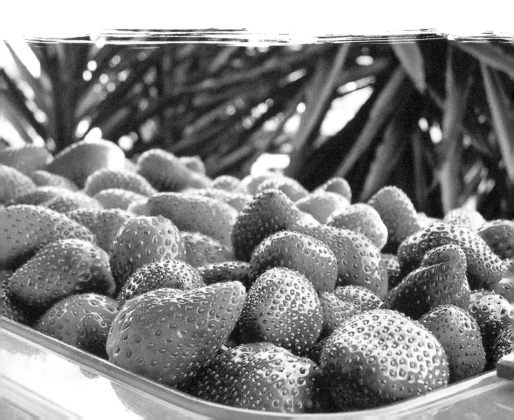

Strawberries are one of the easiest items to freeze. After the vinegar and water rinse previously mentioned, pat your berries dry and spread them on plates or trays that will fit into your freezer. Freeze them overnight and then transfer into freezer-safe containers or bags. If you place berries directly into bags or containers without first freezing them on trays they will clump together and it will be difficult to take out a small serving. When frozen with the tray method the berries will be easy to serve as they won't be stuck together. You can take them out of the bag one at a time.

Parts Used

Obviously, the fruit is edible, but so are the leaves and flowers. I am a big fan of using the entire plant when it is safe to eat it; however, strawberry leaves are very plain and dry. I will toss them into a smoothie or add them to a salad to take advantage of the chlorophyll and B vitamins they contain. They also have a mild diuretic effect. Although the flowers are edible with a pleasant flavor, I prefer not to eat them because I would rather have the berries. On fruiting plants, first the flower forms that gets pollinated by bees, wasps or butterflies. After a successful pollination the fruit starts to form. If the flowers are harvested, there will be no fruit. If you have the opportunity to snack on a strawberry leaf, I encourage you to give it a try; it is good to experience different parts of the plant when you know they are safe to consume.

Nutritional Benefits of Strawberries

Strawberry seeds provide a small amount of protein and fat as well as ellagic acid, a powerful antioxidant and anticancer nutrient. Strawberries are high in vitamin C, folate, manganese and copper, qualifying them as an excellent blood builder.

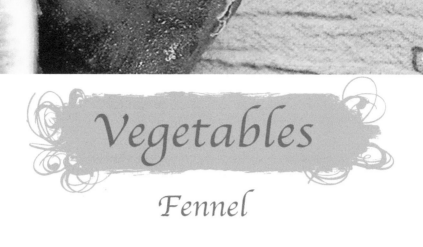

Vegetables

Fennel

This is a fun plant to grow in your own vegetable garden. Not only is it beautiful, it is also very aromatic and has great health benefits. Growing fennel is a wonderful way to be involved with the cycle of life and get something edible from your own backyard.

Fennel is a host plant to black swallowtail butterflies, so we do have to compete with nature to determine who gets to eat first: the black swallowtail caterpillars or us. Black swallowtail butterflies lay their eggs on the tops of fennel plants. When these eggs hatch, tiny caterpillars emerge and eat the plant as their primary food source. Often ten, fifteen or twenty caterpillars can appear overnight. It is fun to watch them grow, but as they mature they eat the fennel plant down to tiny nubs. However, the undamaged bulb underground can still be dug up, prepared and enjoyed as a nice snack or side dish.

If the fennel plant stays in your garden long enough, it will produce delicate, edible flowers that taste just like black licorice candy. If the plant matures even longer, it will produce edible seeds, which you may be accustomed to buying in the store as a culinary spice or tea.

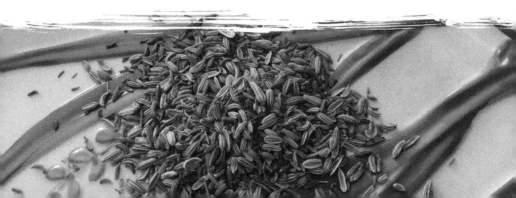

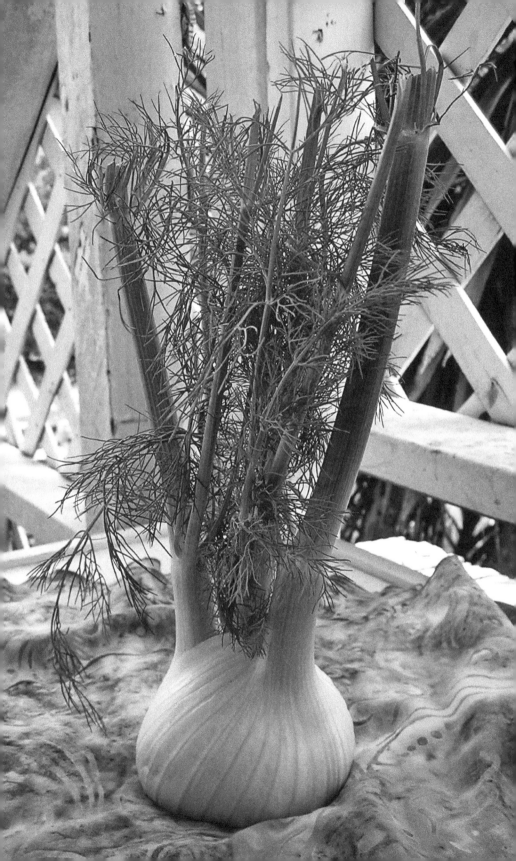

Selecting Fennel

Fresh fennel bulbs are shiny, firm and crisp. Avoid bulbs that are withered or dull looking. Some brown markings are normal, but I don't recommend eating the brown parts.

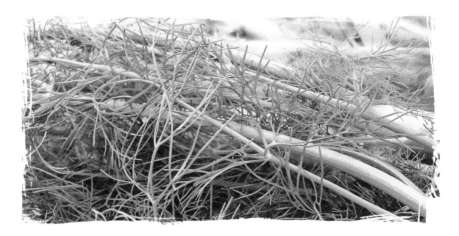

Fennel stems can be compared to celery stalks. The stems should be firm and the feathery leaves perky.

Fennel Seeds

These can be purchased as a bulk herb or a seasoning sold in standard shaker bottles. They can also be purchased in tea bags and easily brewed as a tea to soothe an upset stomach (*see Digestive Tonic Tea recipe, page 148*).

Storing Fennel

If you select a fresh bulb, it will store well for several weeks sealed in a plastic bag in the refrigerator. Since the leaves deteriorate quickly I recommend removing them and eating them immediately. They make a flavorful addition to salads.

Health Benefits of Fennel

Fennel bulbs are high in vitamin C, fiber, potassium and antioxidant compounds. Fennel seeds are considered carminatives, which is a fancy way of saying they relieve gas and indigestion. The seeds can also help increase lactation for breast feeding moms.

It is an eastern tradition to use fennel as a digestive tonic after a large meal. If you have ever eaten at an Indian restaurant, you have likely seen a dish of mysterious looking "after dinner mints" by the door. Try chewing on five or ten fennel seeds or brewing up a hot cup of fennel tea to conclude a large meal.

The entire fennel plant has a distinctive, strong taste that can dominate any dish. I like to pair fennel with orange as these two flavors harmonize well when combined (*see Fennel Orange Salad recipe, page 126*).

Okra

Do you love it or hate it? When you think of okra do memories of slimy, gooey mush come to mind—or, like me, do you look forward to having some in your next meal? Read on for a fresh perspective.

Okra grows prolifically during the summer months in Florida. The plants require very little care and yield enough for me to eat, freeze and have plenty to share with neighbors and friends.

Selecting Okra

The best, fresh-tasting okra comes right off the plant. It starts to wilt and soften within a day or two, which is why most okra is sold frozen. Fresh okra is crisp and crunchy when it is harvested. When selecting okra avoid mold, brown spots and limp pods.

Raw Okra

Raw okra is delicious. Simply wash and dry the pods, cut off the ends and start munching.

Cooked Okra

It seems okra has quite a bad reputation for its slimy texture. This slime (also called mucilage) has medicinal properties. Raw okra does have a small amount of slime, but the more it is handled and cooked, the more mucilage gets released. This is what you might find offensive, but the slime has fantastic health benefits.

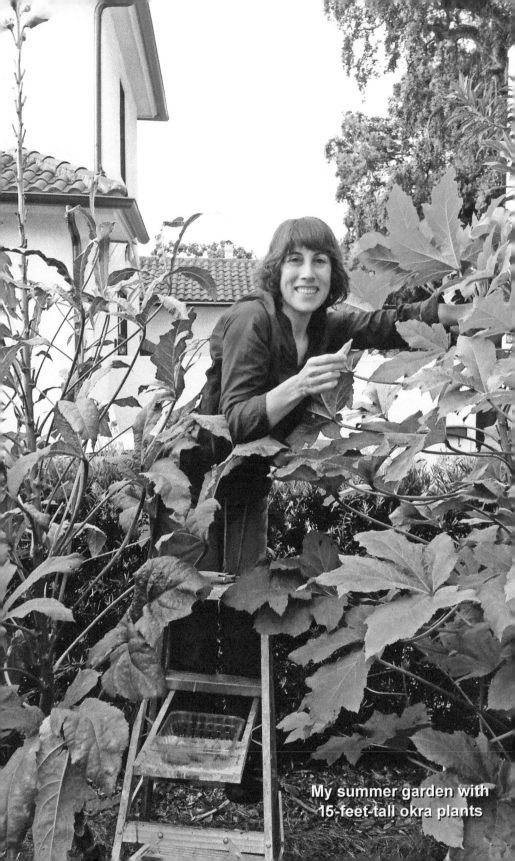

My summer garden with
15-feet-tall okra plants

If you have digestive symptoms such as acid reflux, ulcers or hemorrhoids, this mucilaginous slime is just the natural remedy that can help ease your discomfort. Okra is also beneficial for all of the glands in the body, including your ovaries and thyroid gland. The little seeds inside the okra pods are high in protein and fats, making it a great protein source on a plant-based diet.

Preparing Okra

To reduce the slime, wash the pods and put them into a bowl. Completely cover all the pods with raw apple cider vinegar and let soak for 30 minutes. Remove the pods and rinse them. If you cook the pods whole, without cutting them open, they will not release the mucilage. Alternately a teaspoon of lemon juice added to the cooking water will also reduce the slippery texture.

Health Benefits of Okra

Okra is high in potassium, which is beneficial for your muscles and your heart. Try some okra soup before your next workout (*see Easy Okra Soup recipe, page 133*). The potassium in the okra and the sodium from the salt in this recipe make it a perfect electrolyte replacement drink without all the sugar and chemicals found in packaged sports drinks.

Parsley and Dandelion Greens

When you see a tuft of parsley garnishing on your plate in a restaurant, do you push it aside and eat everything else? This overlooked garnish is loaded with nutrients and deserves to be in the spotlight.

Bitter flavored greens are one of the best digestive tonics. The next time you are at a restaurant try something different: have several sprigs of parsley with your meal to help improve your digestion. Your friends will be glad you did because it is also a great breath freshener!

Incorporating Bitter Greens

Use the leaves and the stems of your parsley and dandelions. The stems of all leafy vegetables are high in silica, a naturally occurring mineral that strengthens your bones, hair and nails. If you are taking nutritional supplements with synthetic silica for this very purpose, consider adding some stems into your diet. The minerals we get through our food are much easier for the body to digest and utilize.

Health Benefits

Fresh parsley has superior medicinal benefits compared to the dried herb found in your kitchen spice rack. Dried parsley has lost much of the folic acid and vitamin C which are present in fresh parsley. It is naturally high in iron, vitamin K and the essential oil limonene, an excellent liver cleanser.

Dandelion is high in calcium, vitamins E, K and folic acid. Dandelion can soothe an upset stomach, minimize intestinal gas and reduce inflammation. It is a natural diuretic that is helpful for swollen ankles or retention of water.

Selecting Parsley and Dandelion

Parsley comes in two varieties, flat leaf and curly leaf. I prefer flat leaf because it is easier to chew, wash, blend and has a better flavor.

Dandelion greens come in several different sizes and varieties. The smaller dandelion leaves tend to be more tender and palatable compared to larger, more mature leaves. The longer the leaves stay on the plant the more bitter they become. You may have some growing wild in your yard. If you spray your yard with any herbicides or pesticides, I don't suggest snacking on wild dandelions sprouting up

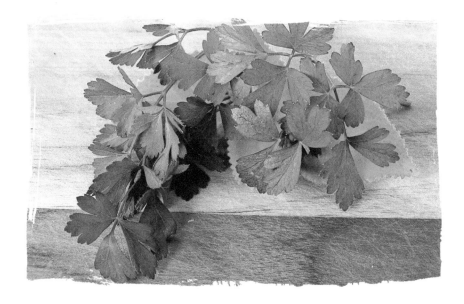

next to your swing set. Support your local economy by purchasing some from a local farm or farmers market. Consider planting some in a pot or start an organic garden. Both of these greens are very easy to grow and require little care once established.

Storing Parsley and Dandelion

Both should be used as soon as possible after being harvested or purchased. Discard any withered or yellowing leaves immediately and store the fresh greens in your refrigerator sealed in a plastic storage bag until you are ready to use them.

Washing Parsley and Dandelion

Place the whole bundle into a bowl of water and swish it around to allow any dirt or sand to come free and sink to the bottom. Repeat this process with clean water until there is no debris at the bottom of the bowl. Take the cleaned greens out of the water and shake them off. Snap the whole bundle into a few pieces and use a salad spinner to remove any unwanted moisture.

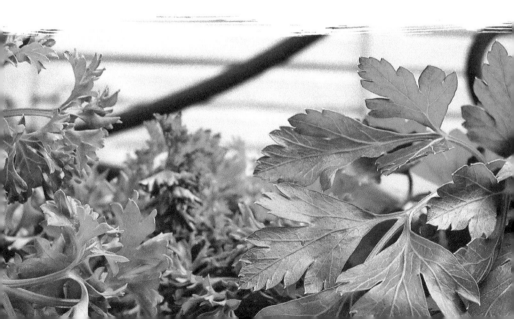

Chopping Your Greens

Place all the greens in a pile on your cutting board and roll them together like a burrito. While you finely chop the stems and leaves take notice of the green pigment that is released onto your knife and cutting board. This is chlorophyll, which is excellent for detoxifying the body and building the blood.

Bitter is Better for Cleansing

These two plants have a strong, bitter flavor, but that is exactly what will detoxify your system. Following a cleansing program is a great way to build up your health reserves, ward off colds and stuffy noses with the change of seasons and turn over a new leaf (*see Super Easy Detox, page 46*).

A few generations ago, it was common knowledge that bitters should accompany a heavy meal. Our grandparents knew this wisdom and practiced it as a way of life. Being old fashioned may be out of style, but not when it comes to bitter greens. Let's continue this natural, sensible practice and bring some bitter flavors back into our diets. Invest in your health today and benefit in the months ahead. This is what preventative self-care is about; take care of your body throughout the year so you are strong and vibrant during the change of seasons.

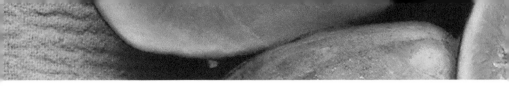

Pumpkin

Are you interested in an eco-friendly way to enjoy Halloween? Celebrate autumn with edible decorations. Now this is a practical way to go green! Decorate your home and doorstep with pumpkins to celebrate the season and then eat up—no waste, no plastic and completely biodegradable.

Due to their orange pigment, pumpkins are naturally high in beta carotene and vitamin A. They are one of the easiest foods for your body to digest, containing rich amounts of fiber and magnesium. They also provide B vitamins, potassium, copper and manganese.

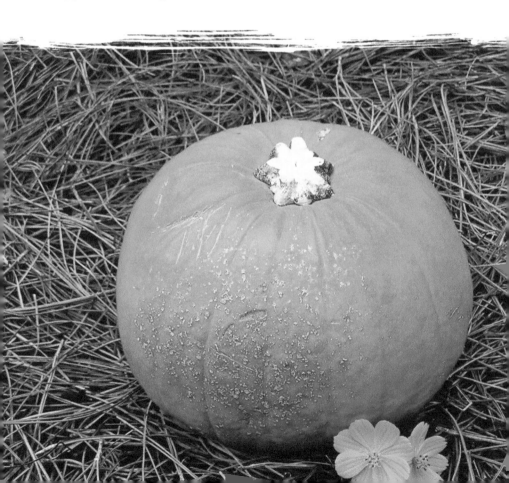

Selecting Pumpkins

All sizes and shapes of pumpkins are edible. My favorite for cooking and baking is the small version called a pie pumpkin. When selecting one to eat, be sure it is heavy compared to other pumpkins the same size. If the pumpkin is light weight, it is dried out on the inside. Heavy pumpkins have moist, dense meat with the highest nutritional benefits.

Storing Pumpkins

Pumpkins should be stored in the refrigerator until ready for use. Just prior to baking, take your pumpkin out of the fridge and let it come to room temperature; this will make it easier to cut open and easier to handle.

Preparation Tip

I have found the best way to cut a pumpkin in half is with the sharp point of a chef's knife. Insert the tip of the knife into the pumpkin just below where the stem attaches and press downward firmly on the handle. Remove the knife and turn the pumpkin over. Repeat this on the other side, just across from your first cut line. If you have followed my suggestions for selecting a pumpkin, it will be fresh and crisp. It will naturally crack open along the cut lines. If you have a tough time getting through the ends with your knife, you can simply cut those off, making it easier to split the pumpkin into two pieces.

Pumpkin Seeds

I prefer to use a spoon with a serrated edge, such as a grapefruit spoon, to scoop out the seeds and inner pulp.

During pumpkin carving rituals, it is common to toast the seeds and eat them. I don't recommend this for two reasons:

- The seeds have a thick and tough outer coating. When chewed up, these have a rugged surface, which is hard on the digestive tract and can cause intestinal disturbance.

- Pumpkin seeds are rich in Omega 3 essential fatty acids. This type of fat is extremely heat sensitive and turns into a trans-fat at just over 100°F. The standard temperature for toasting pumpkin seeds is 250°F. Omega 3 fats are best eaten in a raw, unheated state to get the health benefits.

The green pumpkin seeds available for sale at health food stores are from a different variety of pumpkins; these have the hard outer coating removed. Raw, green pumpkin seeds are high in Omega 3, zinc and protein, making them a great healthy afternoon snack.

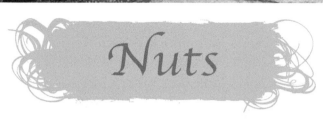

Nuts

Coconuts

Coconuts have been used as a source of food by coastal communities around the world throughout the last several hundred years. These cultures were knowledgeable about selecting edibles for their high nutrient content. We now understand from modern science that coconut contains protein, healthy oils, carbohydrates and high amounts of vitamins and minerals. Eating the inner contents of a coconut is filing and satisfying and comprises a completely balanced meal.

Coconuts naturally contain medium chain triglycerides. Medium chain triglycerides have unique properties compared to all other oils and fats. These are very easy to digest, increase metabolism and help maintain healthy cholesterol levels. Medium chain triglycerides are thermogenic, meaning they have fat burning properties. This can be beneficial as part of a weight loss, diet and exercise program. Medium chain triglycerides are found in fresh coconut meat, coconut oil, coconut butter and shredded coconut.

Coconuts and coconut products can be purchased from grocery stores, health food stores and ethnic markets. There are three varieties to choose from: white, green or brown. White coconuts, known as Thai young coconuts, are stored in a refrigerator. Green and brown coconuts are usually kept at room temperature.

Once the fibrous outer husk is removed, the inner, hard shell can be opened and its treasures revealed. Fresh coconut can be eaten throughout its many stages of maturity. Thai young coconuts are filled with liquid known as coconut water. As the coconut develops, this liquid transforms into a gel. If the coconut continues to grow on the tree, the gel will transform into hard meat.

Depending on the stage of maturity, some coconuts are filled with a large quantity of water, some have gel-like meat and others contain a significant amount of dense meat. Water is found in coconuts that are heavy for their size compared to the other coconuts at the market. Hard meat can be found in coconuts that feel lightweight compared to others the same size. However, the size of a coconut doesn't dictate how much total food it will yield. Huge coconuts can be mostly outer husk

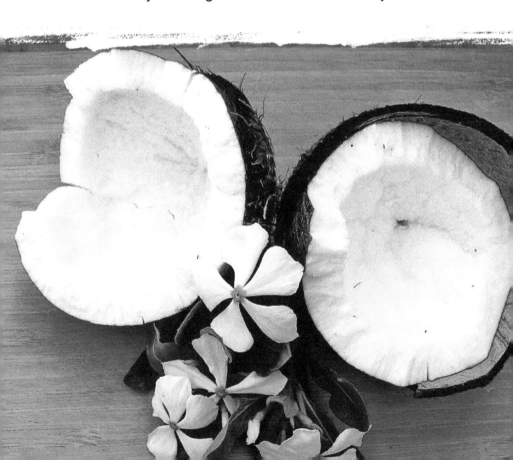

with a tiny, hard, inner shell yielding a very small amount of food. Conversely, small coconuts can be loaded with more than two cups of liquid.

Select only coconuts that look fresh, have no mold on the husk or liquid oozing from the top. I suggest buying several coconuts at a time. When you open them you may discover that they are past their prime and need to be discarded.

When opening all three types of coconuts the water should be drained first. Some coconuts will spray water like a garden hose while getting them open, so it is best to try this outdoors for easier clean up. I like to use a glass one-quart measuring cup to hold the coconut and let the water drain out. Always smell, examine and taste the water for freshness and then open the coconut to get the meat out.

Selecting Dark or Light Brown Coconuts

When shopping for dark or light brown coconuts, only purchase coconuts with no white mold around the three black eyes at the top. Shake the coconut. If it is lightweight and you don't hear liquid sloshing, it is old and will be dry inside. If it is heavy and you don't hear liquid sloshing, take a chance, because it will likely be full of delicious water.

Opening Dark or Light Brown Coconuts

You will need a clean Phillip's screwdriver, a hammer, a measuring cup, a butter knife and a thin kitchen towel. Hammer the screwdriver into each of the black eyes. Turn the coconut upside down and drain the water into the measuring cup. Taste the coconut water to make sure it is fresh; if it has an unpleasant smell, discard it. Place the drained coconut in the freezer for 30 minutes so the meat will be easier to separate from the husk. Remove the coconut from the freezer and wrap it in the kitchen towel. Take it outside, place it onto the cement and whack it with a hammer until it cracks open. Separate the meat from the shell with the butter knife.

Selecting White Coconuts

Select coconuts that are fresh and cold. Avoid green or pink mold inside the plastic wrap. Thai young coconuts should be opened and consumed immediately as they tend to spoil very quickly.

Opening White Coconuts

You will need a wooden spoon, a sharp cleaver, a metal spoon with a serrated edge such as a grapefruit spoon and a large measuring cup.

Turn the coconut so the pointed tip is down and the flat surface is facing up. Drive the handle of the wooden spoon into the center of the flat surface several times until you find the soft spot. Once the spoon handle penetrates the husk, turn it over and place it in the measuring cup to drain. Set the drained coconut on a hard surface, such as cement and then use a cleaver to split it. After it is split, use a grapefruit spoon to scrape out the meat.

Green Coconuts

Opening these requires confidence, skill and accuracy with a machete or a large cleaver. Without skill and accuracy you will likely end up chasing a rolling coconut around your yard with a big knife. Some markets have employees who will open the coconuts for you, just ask. Even if the water has a beige or grey tinge, it is still fresh and drinkable.

Although it is quite a treat to eat a coconut right off the palm tree, you can enjoy the luxury and health benefits of coconuts right in your own kitchen. Coconut products are great alternatives for those on gluten-free or dairy-free diets. For something different, try delicious treats such as coconut ice cream and other desserts now being widely distributed.

Coconut Oil

Just as olive oil is extracted from olives, coconut oil is extracted from coconut meat. It is a liquid when it is 78°F or warmer and solid when it is below 78°F. Its molecular structure is stable up to 400°F, which makes it a great oil for cooking and baking.

Coconut oil is delicious in smoothies and salad dressings. It can be used as a thickener in puddings, sorbets or dairy-free ice creams. Coconut oil is rapidly absorbed by the body and is one of the best oils to eat for this reason. Coconut oil can also be used topically to soothe dry skin instead of lotion.

Coconut Butter

Just like peanuts get creamed into peanut butter, coconut butter is made from creamed coconut meat. Similar to coconut oil, the butter is liquid above 78°F. It is thicker than coconut oil and can be drizzled onto fruits such as papaya or eaten with a spoon right from the jar.

To liquefy hardened coconut oil or butter (necessary in the winter months): put a little into a pan and turn the burner on the lowest setting. It will be melted in just a few minutes.

Coconut Water

Coconut water has the highest mineral content and lowest sugar content when taken from fresh coconuts. Packaged coconut water is usually pasteurized, which is a heating and sterilization process that changes the nutritional profile and flavor. It doesn't compare to the fresh taste, but fortunately it is accessible and available at health food stores, and many Jamaican and Spanish markets. Coconut water is refreshing on a hot day, after working out or sweating, and is an exceptional source of electrolytes. It is delicious as is or can be used in smoothies.

Coconut Milk

Coconut milk is sometimes confused with coconut water. These are actually two different things. Coconut milk is coconut meat blended with water and is a common ingredient in recipes with an Asian influence.

Shredded, Dried or Desiccated Coconut

These are different names for the same product. This is coconut meat (sometimes called copra) that has been dried and shredded. It can be purchased in most grocery stores in the baking aisle and sprinkled on top of desserts, made into macaroons and used in Asian recipes.

Coconut Flour

Dried coconut with the oil extracted yields flour, which can be used when baking. Unlike all other types of flour, this absorbs every liquid added to it except coconut oil. This completely changes the ratio of dry to liquid ingredients so it cannot be easily substituted in traditional recipes. There is an art to baking with coconut flour and it is necessary to follow a recipe. This flour is great for gluten-free diets or adding a different flavor and experience to baking.

Coconut Vinegar

This is made from fermented coconut. It can be used in salad dressings and marinades. It is a powerful digestive stimulant and skin tonic.

With so many products now available, it will be easy for you to get acquainted with the health benefits coconuts can offer. Coconut products taste delicious on their own and add wonderful texture to many dishes. No matter how you cut it, smash it or chase it around your yard—coconut is loaded with nutrients and excellent for your health.

Pecans

Selecting Pecans in the Shell

All nuts are high in healthy oils that can go rancid quickly. Buying pecans still in the shell will ensure that the flavor is good and the oils are still stable. As soon as the nut shells are cracked open, the oils start to break down. The shell acts as somewhat of a preservative for the natural oils.

When buying pecans in a package or from a bulk bin, choose only those that look fresh and clean. Shelled pecans can go rancid much more quickly than pecans still in the shell, but proper storage will help preserve them longer. Select pecans that look undamaged without crumbs in the bulk bin or package.

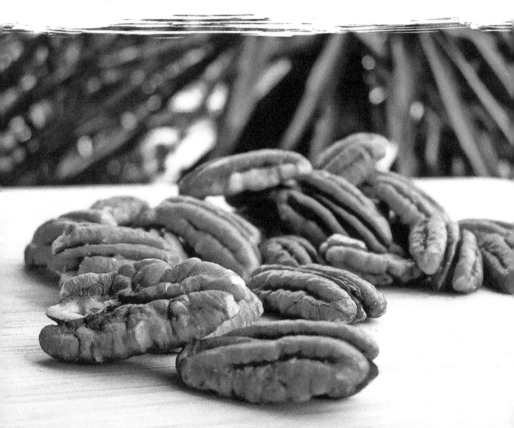

Storing Pecans

Pecans should be stored in a sealed bag or container. They can be refrigerated or frozen. Simply let them thaw to room temperature prior to consuming.

Nutritional Benefits of Pecans

Fresh pecans are an excellent source of protein and essential fatty acids (Omega 3 and Omega 6), which have anti-inflammatory properties. Pecans are naturally high in thiamin, which is part of the vitamin B complex as well as manganese and copper.

"For years I struggled with chronic pain, depression and food allergies. I tried everything and was on a ton of supplements. After months of taking the supplements I realized that I wasn't getting much better. I heard about Samadhi's Sustainable Nutrition class and decided to attend. I learned so much about food and how it can help you. I took the summer and really focused on the foods that were beneficial for my health problems. I even kept the information I received from the class on the kitchen counter and referred to it on a regular basis. I can honestly say that it changed me. My pain went away and I was no longer depressed. I needed the real nutrients from real food. Since then I have incorporated what I learned into my daily life and I am so grateful for the knowledge."

—L. P., Lake Mary, Florida

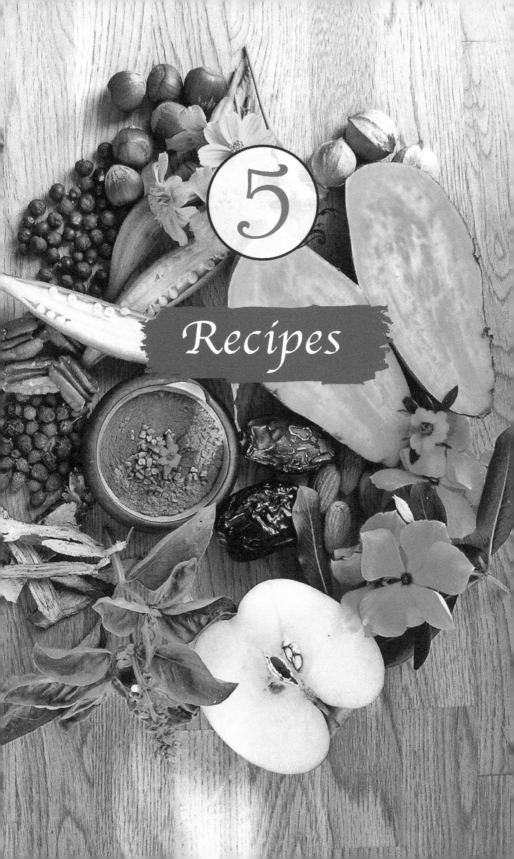

5

Recipes

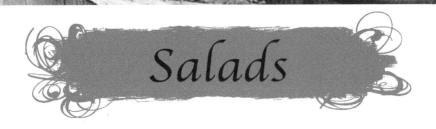

Salads

Festive Fennel Orange Salad

2 bulbs of fennel,
chopped

3 medium oranges,
peeled

1 bundle spinach,
washed and chopped

Spread chopped spinach onto a dinner plate. Mix fennel and orange in a bowl and set aside.

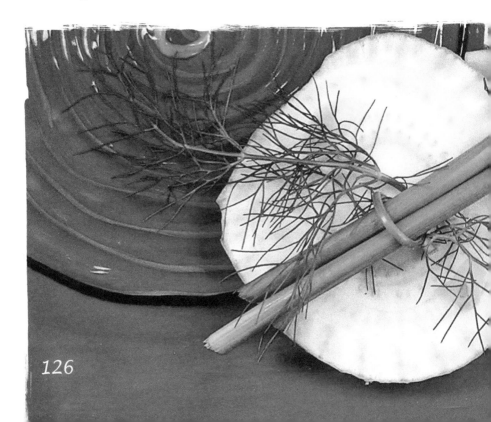

Dressing

4 tablespoons cold pressed, extra virgin olive oil	¼ cup orange juice
	1 teaspoon orange zest
1 tablespoon lemon juice	pinch of salt

Mix all ingredients in a bowl until the salt dissolves. Pour dressing over the fennel and orange mixture and toss until ingredients are evenly distributed. Spoon entire mixture over the spinach and top with a few fennel leaves.

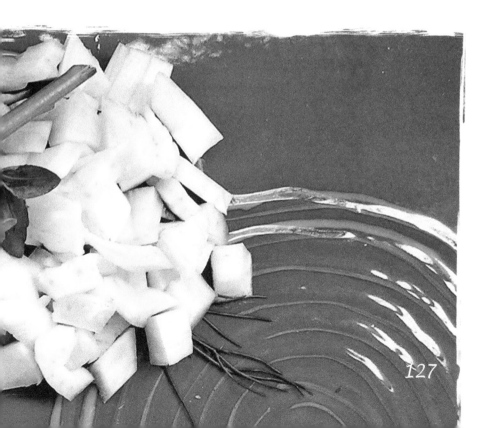

Savory Salad

2-4 cups baby lettuce

1 scallion, chopped

1 rib of celery, chopped

3 radishes, chopped

2 tablespoons extra virgin, cold pressed olive oil

2 teaspoons raw apple cider vinegar

1 teaspoon ground flax seeds

½ cucumber, peeled and chopped

Place all of your prepared vegetables and toppings into a large bowl, toss and eat.

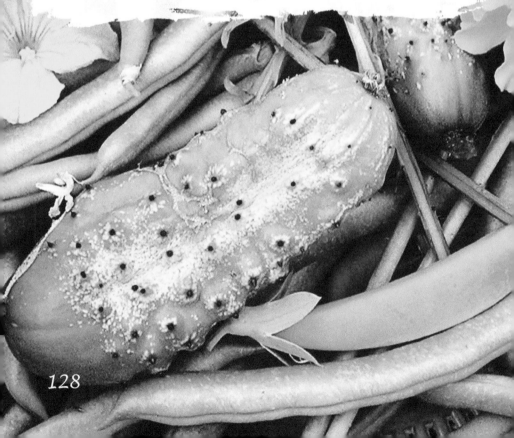

Liver and Gallbladder Cleanser Salad

½ bundle of parsley, chopped

½ bundle of dandelion greens, chopped

3 tablespoons raw pumpkin seeds

2 teaspoons ground flax seeds

5 cherry tomatoes sliced in half

3 tablespoons extra virgin, cold pressed olive oil

lemon juice to taste

pinch of salt

Arrange the greens on your plate and top with the cherry tomatoes. In a small bowl, mix the pumpkin seeds, flax seeds, olive oil, lemon juice and pinch of salt. Garnish the salad with this mixture.

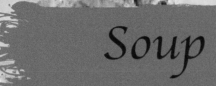

Soup

Vegetarian Squash Soup

1 small acorn squash

1 cup raw cashews (soaked in water for 2 hours)

3 tablespoons raw honey or brown rice syrup

½ teaspoon nutmeg

1 teaspoon ginger powder

1 teaspoon salt

½ tsp black pepper

shredded coconut (unsweetened)

water

Preheat oven to 400°F. Cut your squash in half and remove the seeds. Place the halves open side down in a glass baking dish. Bake for about 30 minutes or until a fork easily punctures through the skin and all the meat.

After baking, scoop the meat out and add it to your blender with cashews and just enough water to turn the blades. Pureé until smooth (adding more water if necessary). Add nutmeg, ginger, honey or brown rice syrup, salt and pepper. Blend for 1 more minute to mix in seasonings.

Top with shredded coconut and serve.

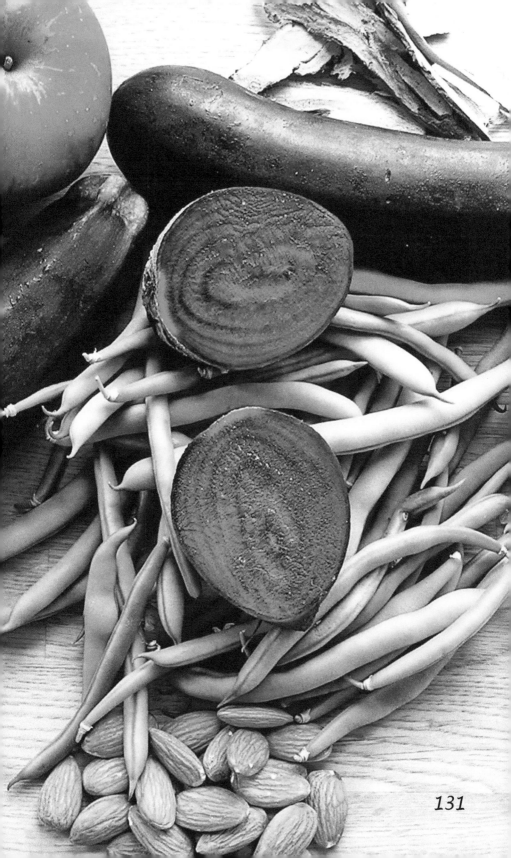

Tomato Soup

- 3 large tomatoes
- 2 tablespoons extra virgin, cold pressed olive oil
- 1 teaspoon chia seeds
- 1 tablespoon turmeric root powder
- 2 cloves of garlic, peeled and crushed
- 1 teaspoon raw honey or brown rice syrup
- pinch of salt

Put all the ingredients into your blender and pureé until smooth. For a gazpacho variation, add a splash of vinegar, top with chopped onions and sliced cucumber. You can have this soup raw (right from the blender) or if you prefer you can warm it in a saucepan on the stove.

Easy Okra Soup

6 fresh or frozen okra pods	1 quart water
	pinch of salt

Wash and cut off the ends of the pods. Cut each pod in half lengthwise. Boil 1 quart water. Add okra and cook for 10 minutes. Add a pinch of salt and consume the whole dish as a soup. See page 105 for cooking tips to reduce the slippery texture.

Okra Electrolyte Drink

Strain the cooked okra over a bowl. Save the liquid and discard the solids. Add a pinch of salt to your taste preference and drink the broth.

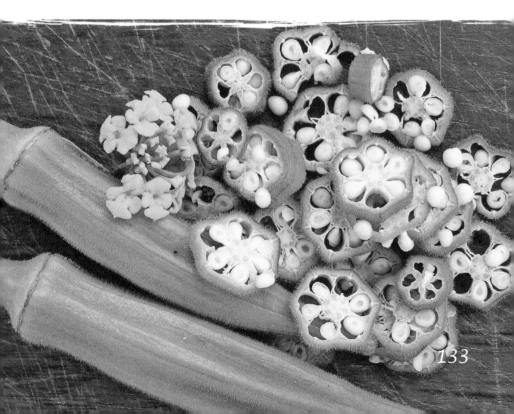

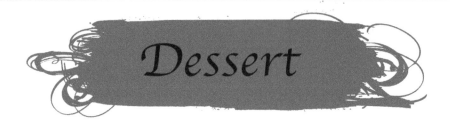

Dessert

Mango Lime Sorbet

3 ripe mangoes

1 banana

¼ cup lime juice

½ cup shredded coconut

pinch of salt

water (if needed to turn the blades of the blender)

Cut the flesh from the mangoes and discard the pits and peels. Put all the ingredients in a blender. After adding the lime juice, if more liquid is required, add water to just barely cover the solid ingredients. Blend until completely smooth. Pour into freezer-safe containers or an ice pop mold. Freeze for about 6 hours.

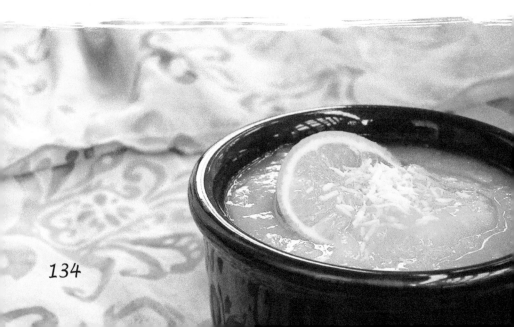

Persimmon Pudding

3 ripe bananas

1 tablespoon raw honey or brown rice syrup

4 ripe persimmons, peeled

1 teaspoon alcohol-free vanilla flavoring

Add all ingredients to the blender and liquefy until smooth. Pour into small dessert bowls. Place the mixture in the freezer, and chill for 45 minutes, then serve.

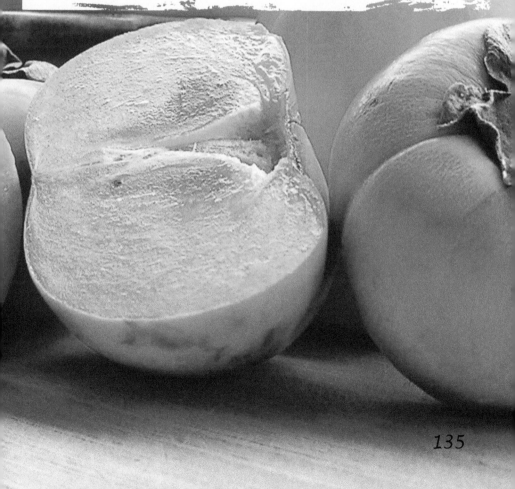

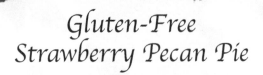

Gluten-Free
Strawberry Pecan Pie

The Crust

- 2 cups raw, shelled pecans
- 2 cups Medjool dates (pitted)
- 2 tablespoons coconut oil
- ½ teaspoon salt
- pinch of cinnamon

Grease an 8" pie pan with a light coating of coconut oil.

In a food processor using the metal S-blade, process all ingredients together until the mixture crumbles.

Press it into the pie pan and set aside.

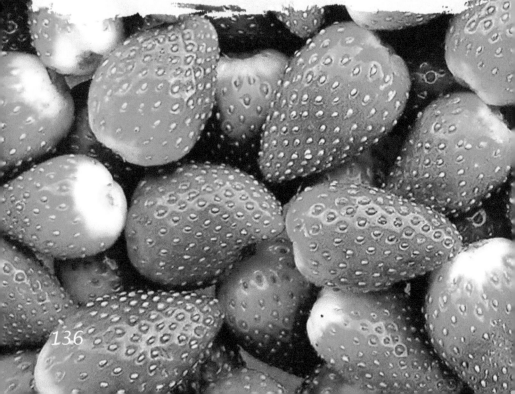

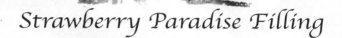

Strawberry Paradise Filling

3 cups fresh or frozen strawberries

¾ cup raw cashews

3 tablespoons chia seeds

1 teaspoon salt

3 tablespoons raw honey or brown rice syrup

2 teaspoons alcohol-free vanilla flavoring

water

Add all ingredients to blender and barely cover with water. Blend until smooth.

Pour mixture into the crust and place in freezer until it firms up (several hours).

Garnish the pie with sliced strawberries before serving.

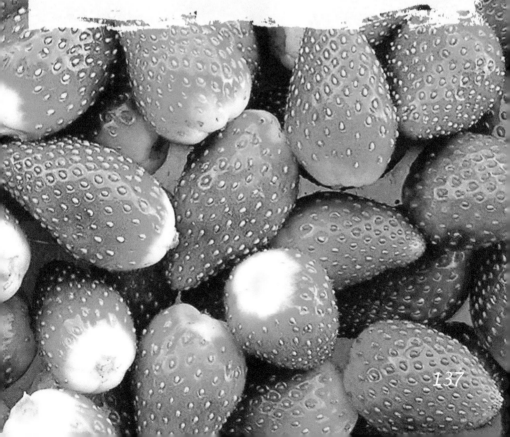

Raw Halvah

10 oz. raw tahini (sesame seed paste)

6 oz. raw honey or brown rice syrup

4 oz. melted coconut oil

Add tahini, melted coconut oil and honey or brown rice syrup into a bowl. Stir with a large spoon to evenly distribute the mixture and then spread on a piece of parchment paper. Slide the parchment paper on top of a cutting board or plate and freeze for 2 hours. Cut into pieces and eat immediately upon thawing. Store the unused portions in the freezer in a container layered with parchment paper to keep it separated.

Testimonial

"Our magazine readers love Samadhi's monthly articles which encourage us to eat seasonal foods and inform about their many health benefits. Thanks to her, I now have new favorites which include mangoes, persimmons and—even okra. Yum! Her recipes are easy and fun to make. I'm always excited to try them all!"

—*Margaret Jones Bertone, Publisher*
Natural Awakenings Magazine
Orlando/Central FL Edition

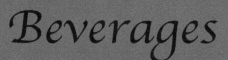

Beverages

Almond Milk

1 cup raw almonds (soaked 8 hours or overnight)	pinch of salt
2 cups water	raw honey or brown rice syrup to taste

Rinse almonds after soaking and discard soaking water. Place almonds, clean water and dash of salt in blender and liquefy. Alternately, you can boil some water and drop the almonds into it for one minute. Skins can be slipped off and discarded and nuts can be blended into milk without soaking.

Strain through a nylon paint strainer bag that can be purchased at a hardware store in the paint department for about $1. Put the mix into a bag, squeeze thoroughly over a large bowl to extract the milk from the pulp.

Add a bit of honey or brown rice syrup if you prefer a sweeter taste or use as is. You can drink the blended mixture with the pulp instead of straining it.

If you extract the pulp it can be used in pie crusts, cookies and breads. Freeze it for possible future use. Milk keeps fresh for up to two days in the fridge; store in tightly sealed jar or container. Other raw nuts and seeds can be substituted for the almonds.

Cashew Milk

1 cup raw cashews	½ banana
2 cups water	½ teaspoon alcohol-free vanilla flavoring
pinch of salt	

Soak the cashews in water (to soften them) for two hours prior to making the recipe. Drain the soaking water and rinse the cashews. Add cashews and 2 cups of clean water; blend until smooth. Add salt, banana and vanilla to your taste preference and blend.

If you want thicker milk, use less water or more nuts. If you want thinner milk, add more water. Store in the refrigerator in a jar or container with a tight-fitting lid and use within two days.

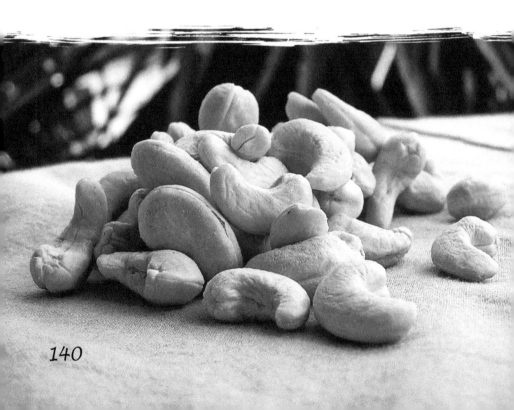

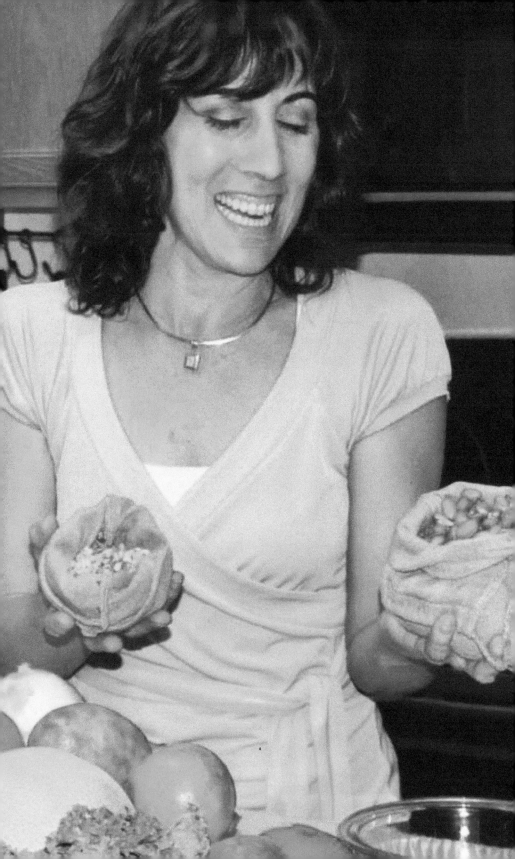

Spicy Lemonade

juice of 1 lemon	1/8 teaspoon turmeric root powder
1/8 teaspoon cayenne pepper	2 cups of water
1 teaspoon chia seeds	1 teaspoon raw honey or brown rice syrup

Add water to a wide mouth bowl. Roll your lemon on the counter or cutting board to loosen the flesh and then slice it in half. Place a mesh strainer over the top of the bowl and squeeze the lemon over the strainer to catch the seeds. Add the rest of the ingredients to the liquid mixture, stir vigorously and drink immediately.

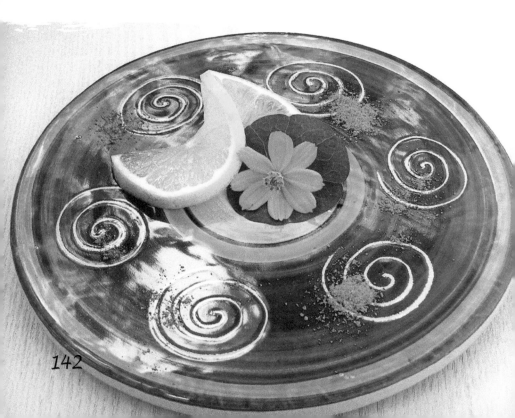

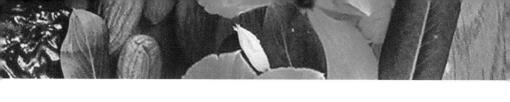

Green Smoothie #1

large handful of spinach

½ cup fresh or frozen
  blueberries

1 banana

8 ounces water

1 teaspoon turmeric root
powder

1 teaspoon flax seeds

1 teaspoon chia seeds

Put all the ingredients into your blender and cover them with water. Blend until smooth.

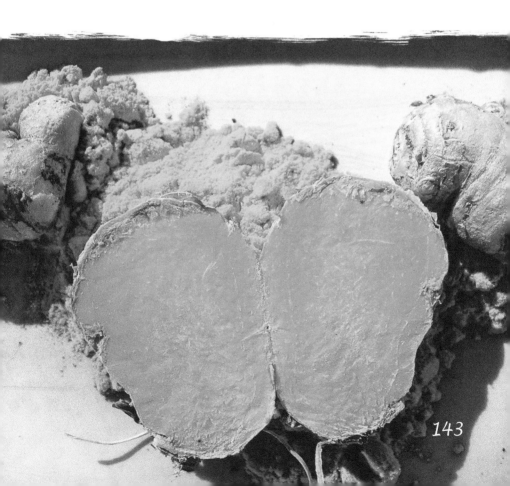

Green Smoothie #2

1 banana   2 cups parsley, chopped
juice of 1 whole orange

Blend the banana and orange juice together until smooth. Add parsley and liquefy for 2-4 minutes.

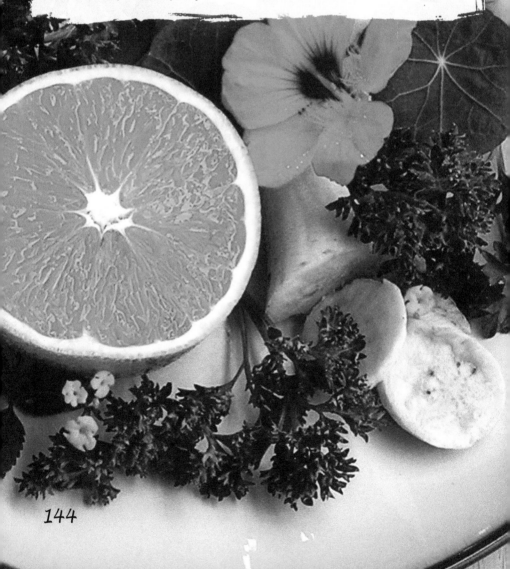

Green Energy Booster

½ bundle parsley, chopped

½ bundle dandelion greens, chopped

1 tablespoon fresh garlic, chopped

2 tablespoons lemon juice

1 quart water

Place all of the chopped greens, lemon juice and water into a bowl. After soaking for 1 hour, strain the solids and sip the chlorophyll rich liquid. The solids can be mixed into a salad or eaten as a side dish.

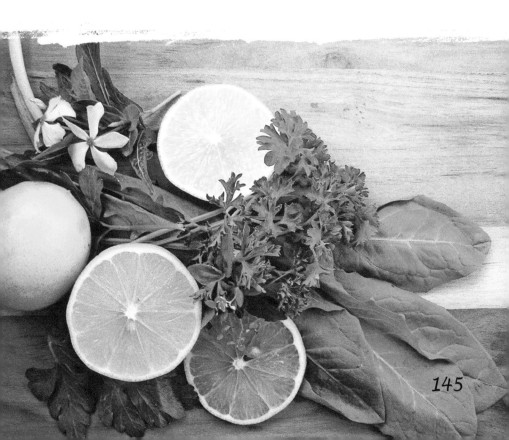

Blood Builder Green Drink

2 cups dandelion greens, chopped

1 cup fresh or frozen cherries, pitted

1 orange, peeled and deseeded

1 banana

water

Put cherries into your blender and let them thaw for 15 minutes. Place orange and peeled banana in the blender. Cover all the fruit with just enough water to rotate the blade of the blender when you turn it on. Blend until creamy. Add dandelion greens and liquefy until it is a smooth consistency.

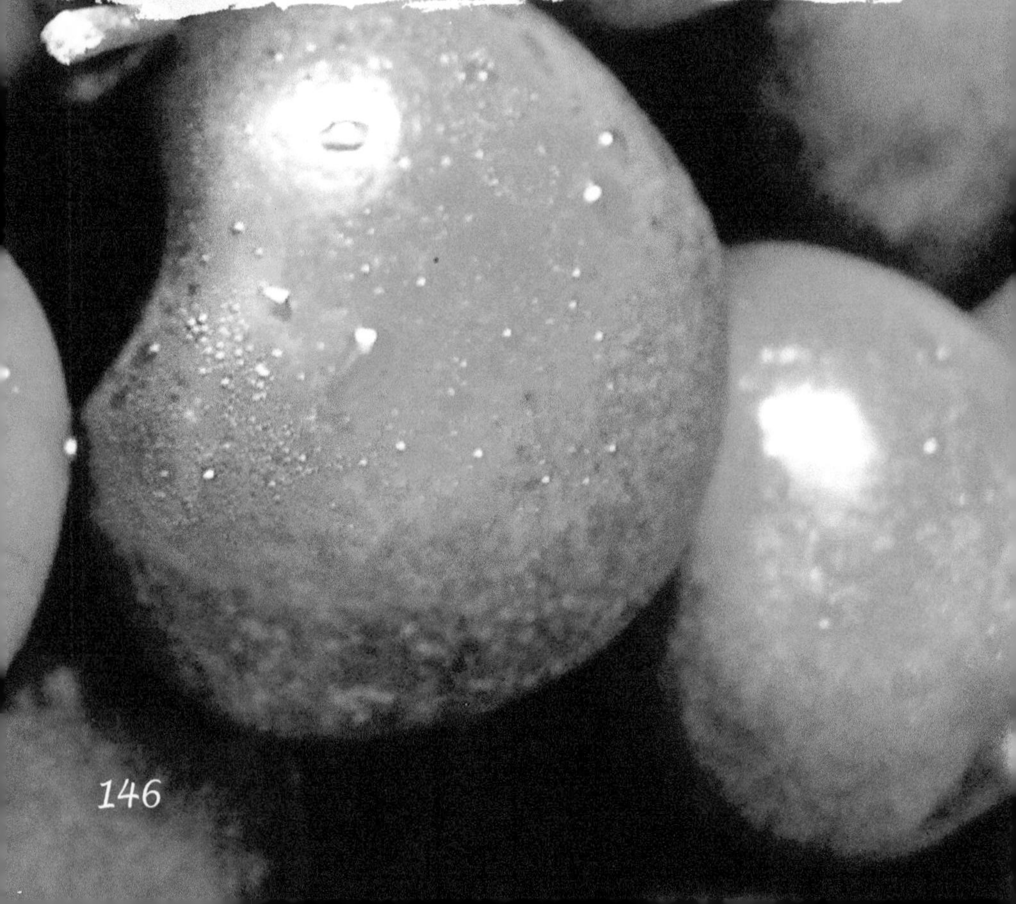

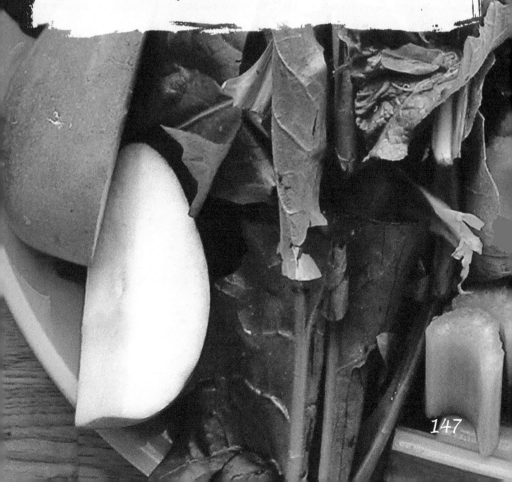

Bittersweet Green Drink

1 bundle of parsley, chopped

1 bundle of dandelion greens, chopped

2 red apples

1 quart water

Core apples and cut them into small chunks. Add 1 quart water and apple chunks to your blender and liquefy these ingredients first. Add the chopped greens to your blended apple mixture and liquefy for 2-4 minutes. Drink the mixture immediately.

Digestive Tonic Tea

1 tablespoon fennel
  seeds, ground or
  crushed

dash of cinnamon
  powder

2 tablespoons
  orange juice

¼ teaspoon orange zest

1 quart water

Bring all ingredients to a boil and let simmer for 2 minutes. Strain and serve. This can be enjoyed hot or cold and sweetened with honey.

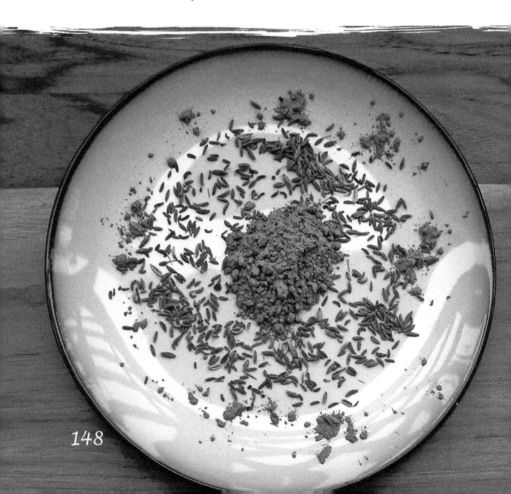

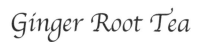

Ginger Root Tea

3-inch piece of fresh,
  peeled ginger root

1 quart of water

1 tablespoon raw
  honey or brown rice
  syrup

Boil the ginger root in water for 5 minutes then let it cool. Serve with a touch of honey or brown rice syrup if you prefer a sweeter beverage.

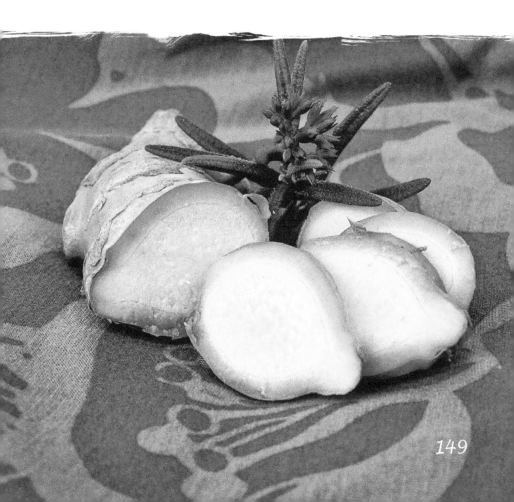

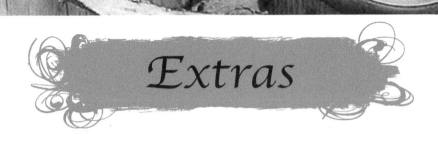

Extras

Pickled Beets

3 medium-sized beets	2 cups water
2 cups raw apple cider vinegar	pinch of salt

Peel and slice the beets into bite sized pieces. Place the beets in a 1 quart glass jar. Put in a pinch of salt. Fill jar with apple cider vinegar half way to the top of the beets and add water to cover the top of the beets. Tightly close the lid on the jar and refrigerate.

Within one week the beets will be pickled and ready to eat. The longer they sit in the vinegar, the softer they become. Eat within one month.

Serve as a side dish or as a garnish on a salad.

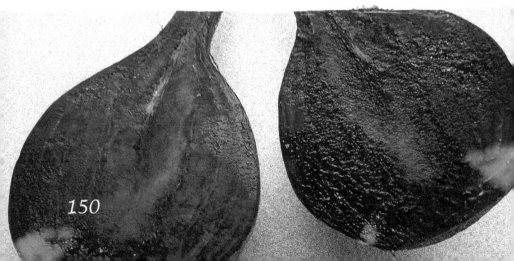

Gluten-Free Hot Cereal

1/3 cup total of a mixture of dry buckwheat, quinoa and millet	1 1/3 cup water

Grind the above grain mix in a coffee grinder until you have a fine powder consistency.

In a small pot bring water to a boil. Add the ground grain mixture and stir constantly with a fork for several minutes until it starts to thicken. Turn the burner off and continue stirring for several minutes. The cereal will continue to thicken.

Serve with ground nuts, seeds and fruit of your choice.

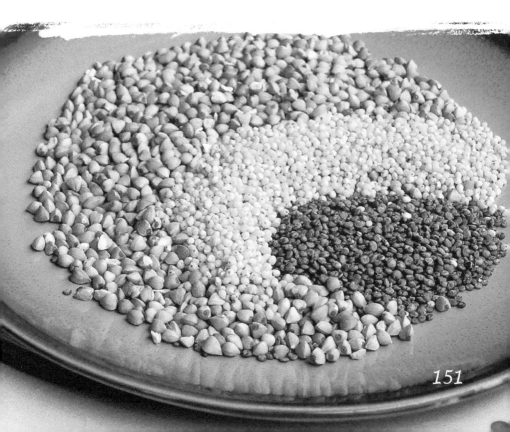

Raw Wilted Greens

1 bundle any variety of kale

1 bundle spinach

juice of 1 small orange

1 teaspoon salt

Wash, dry and chop the greens into bite sized pieces. Put them into a bowl with a few spoonfuls of orange juice and salt. Gently toss to mix the ingredients together. Let this mixture sit for 10 minutes. Using your hands, massage the greens until they turn dark green and start to wilt.

Serve as a side dish or use as the base for a salad and top with other vegetables, raw nuts and seeds. For more dressing add the remaining orange juice.

Kale and Spinach Chips

Follow the Raw Wilted Greens recipe, omitting the orange juice. Use parchment paper to line a cookie sheet or baking dish. After massaging salt into the kale and spinach, spread the wilted greens onto the parchment paper and bake at 250°F until crisp and crunchy.

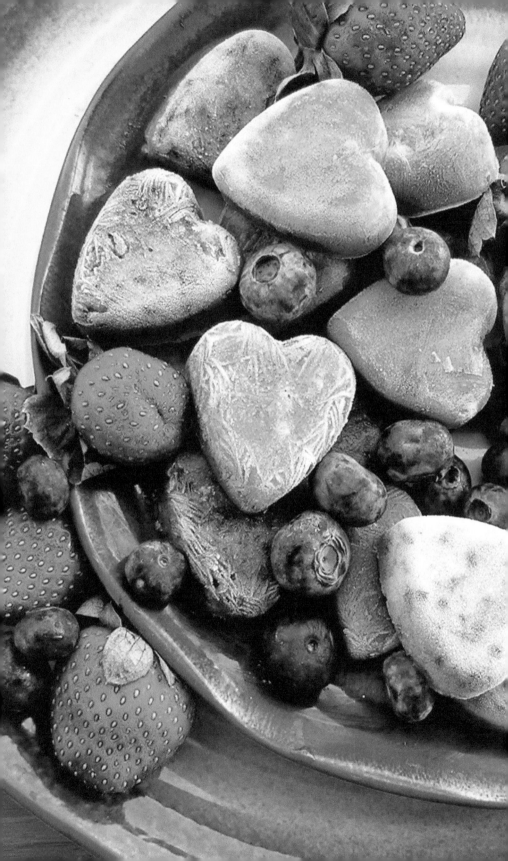

About the Author

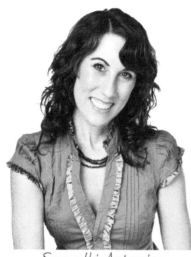

Samadhi Artemisa

Samadhi Artemisa has been a Florida-licensed Acupuncture Physician (AP2278) and Diplomate of Oriental Medicine (NCCAOM 30009) since 2006.

She graduated Cum Laude with her Master's degree in Oriental Medicine and Bachelor's degree in Professional Health Studies from Florida College of Integrative Medicine in 2006.

She is a certified Iridologist through the International Iridology Practitioner's Association (2013), The International Institute of Iridology (2008) and the Bernard Jensen Institute (2007).

Samadhi has a private practice at InJoy Healthcare in Orlando, Florida (established 2007).

Her monthly health column has appeared in "A Better You" of the *Orlando Sentinel* newspaper since 2012 and she has been a speaker on healthy eating and healthy living since 2010.

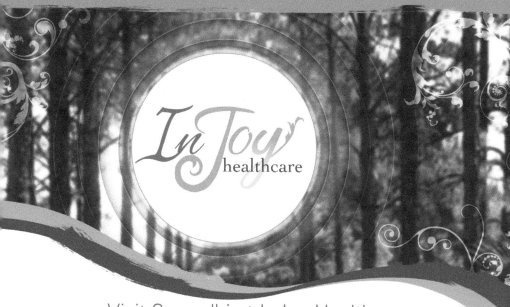

Visit Samadhi at InJoy Healthcare

Get Healthy Feel Great

acupuncture ❧ iridology ❧ nutrition
Holistic Healthcare that Works

www.InJoyHealthcare.com

📍 5021 Eggleston Avenue Ste. C • Orlando, FL 32804

✉ Samadhi@InJoyHealthcare.com 📞 407-252-1397

Healthy Eating Healthy Living Healthy YOU   **157**

Glossary

Acupressure—a way of applying pressure to acupuncture points on the body without using needles.

Bioflavonoids—part of the vitamin C complex, including hesperidin, quercetin and rutin. These naturally occur in many foods and are also sold as a supplement.

Carminative—herb or food that relieves intestinal gas, cramping, bloating and discomfort of the digestive tract.

Casein—protein found in milk.

Chlorophyll—a green pigment found in all leafy green vegetables that helps the plant absorb light during photosynthesis.

Chrysalis—the second stage in the life cycle of a butterfly. The mature caterpillar hangs upside down encased in a chrysalis.

Copra—dried coconut meat.

Dysglycemia—irregular blood sugar levels.

Ellagic acid—an anticancer substance found in strawberry seeds and other foods.

Germination—the sprouting of a seed.

Gluten—a protein in many grains. When glutinous grains, such as wheat, are used to make dough, it is the gluten that gives the elastic, stretchy and sticky texture.

GMO—an acronym for Genetically Modified Organism.

Holistic—an approach to looking at the body as a whole, recognizing interdependence of its parts.

Hybrid—a mixture of plant characteristics to create a new, stronger, disease-resistant, and often, seedless plant.

Instar—the first stage in the life cycle of a caterpillar as it goes through metamorphosis into a butterfly. During this stage, the caterpillar eats, grows and sheds its skin several times.

Insulin resistance—a condition in which the body stops responding to insulin (a hormone secreted by the pancreas in response to consuming carbohydrates).

Iridology—a tool used for looking at the iris of the eye. Each iris is made of over 20,000 nerve endings, which make a map of the genetic traits.

Iris—the colored part of the eyes (blue, hazel or brown).

Limonene—an essential oil found in citrus peels and many other foods and herbs. This oil gives off the wonderful aroma from citrus peels.

Medium chain triglyceride—a type of fat naturally occurring in coconut. Because of the unique molecular structure, it is more easily digested than many other types of fats.

Meridian—an energy pathway in the body, similar to the latitude and longitude lines on the Earth. These are invisible lines; you don't see them when you cross the equator yet they are used for navigation. The foundation of acupuncture is based on using these lines to restore balance in the body.

Mucilage—a slimy, therapeutic secretion from foods such as okra, flax seeds and chia seeds.

Omega 3, 6 and 9 essential fatty acids—technical names for the molecular structures of the fatty acids that naturally occur in many nuts, seeds and fish.

Pasteurization—a process of heating food at high enough temperatures for a duration of time to kill microorganisms that can cause fermentation or spoilage.

Perfluorinated chemicals (PFCs)—chemicals used in stain resistant coatings and nonstick coatings that repel grease and water.

Qi—the energy that moves through the meridians of the body. In Chinese Medicine, blocked or stagnant Qi is the root cause of pain and other organ imbalances in the body. Acupuncture can help create a free flow of this energy.

rBGH—(recombinant Bovine Growth Hormone) a genetically modified hormone that increases milk production in cows.

Saturated fat—fats such as coconut oil and butter that are solid at room temperature.

Smoke point—when an oil or fat is heated, this is the temperature at which the molecular structure breaks down.

Thermogenic—a substance, such as coconut oil, which speeds up the metabolism and burns fat.

Unsaturated fat—also known as oils that are liquid at room temperature.

Resources

"A Better You," the *Orlando Sentinel* newspaper
www.OrlandoSentinel.com/ABetterYou

A Natural Farm and Education Center
www.ANaturalFarm.com

Center for Food Safety
www.CenterForFoodSafety.org

Dr. Ellen Tart-Jensen
www.BernardJensen.com

Samadhi's Website
InJoy Healthcare
www.InJoyHealthcare.com

Environmental Working Group
www.EWG.org

Florida Board of Acupuncture
www.FloridasAcupuncture.gov

Florida U-Pick Farms
www.PickYourOwn.org/FL.htm

Florida Vegetable Gardening Guide
www.Edis.ifas.Ufl.edu/vh021

Institute for Responsible Technology
www.ResponsibleTechnology.org

International Iridology Practitioners Association
www.iridologyassn.org

Lake Meadow Naturals Farm
www.LakeMeadowNaturals.com

Local Roots
www.LocalRootsDistribution.com

Matt D. Smith, Graphic Artist: MDSmith Design
www.MDSmithDesign.com

Michael Cairns, Photographer: Wet Orange Studio
www.MichaelCairns.com

National Certification Commission for Acupuncture and Oriental Medicine
www.nccaom.org

Natural Awakenings, *Orlando/Central Florida Edition*
www.NaturalAwakeningsMag.com

Non-GMO Shopping Guide
www.NonGMOShoppingGuide.com

Non-GMO Project
www.NonGMOProject.org

Organic Consumers Association
www.OrganicConsumers.org

Patricia Charpentier, Editor: Writing Your Life
www.WritingYourLife.org

The information in this book began as published articles written by Samadhi Artemisa and are used with permission from the *Orlando Sentinel* newspaper, *Natural Awakenings Magazine*, *Simple Living Institute* and *Velocity Magazine*. The contents have been adjusted for consistency and flow within the context of the book.

"A Better You," Orlando Sentinel Newspaper

"Silky Smooth Skin with Body Brushing: The Secret to a Youthful, Healthy Glow," March 2013

"Spring Detox: A Jumpstart to Renewed Health," April 2013

"Natural Remedies for an Easy Pregnancy," May 2013

"Uncover the Secrets to Achieving Your Ideal Weight," June 2013

"How to Choose Healthy Foods for You and Your Family," July 2013

"Stop Counting Sheep and Get the Beauty Rest You Need, Naturally," August 2013

"Keep Your Family Healthy with Acupuncture," September 2013

"Nutrition and Iridology: A Holistic Look," October 2013

"3 Easy Steps to Becoming a Local Foodie," November 2013

"Metamorphosis—Becoming the New You," December 2013

"Fit Into Your Skinny Jeans and Never Overeat Again," January 2014

Natural Awakenings Magazine, Central Florida Edition

"Cleansing and Detoxification," July 2012

"Go Green and Eat Your Greens: Sustainable Nutrition for You and Our Planet," January 2013

"Eat Seasonally, Eat Locally, Eat Healthy: Mangoes and Okra," August 2013

"Eat Seasonally, Eat Locally, Eat Healthy: Bitter Is Better for Cleansing, Parsley and Dandelion," September 2013

"Eat Seasonally, Eat Locally, Eat Healthy: Persimmons and Pumpkins," October 2013

"Eat Seasonally, Eat Locally, Eat Healthy: Oranges and Fennel," November 2013

"Eat Seasonally, Eat Locally, Eat Healthy: Pecans and Strawberries," December 2013

"Get the Skinny on Fats and Oils," January 2014

Simple Living Institute Blog

"Keeping Genetically Modified Foods Off of Your Plate," September 2012

Velocity Magazine (no longer published)

"For Your Eating InJoy-ment: Recipes," March, 2014

We Care Magazine (no longer published)

"Taking the Mystery Out of Coconuts," September 2010

Medical Disclaimer

The author of this book is a licensed Acupuncture Physician in Florida (AP2278) and Diplomate in Oriental Medicine (NCCAOM 30009). The descriptions of health-supporting behaviors and activities set forth herein are reflective of the adjunctive therapies and diagnostic techniques of traditional Chinese medical concepts and modern Oriental medical techniques including iridology, lifestyle and nutritional counseling, and the use of herbs and dietary supplements to promote and support good health.

Reading the information in this book and/or incorporating any of the techniques, supplements or advice discussed herein does not create any professional relationship between the reader and Samadhi Artemisa or any other contributor to the book.

The contents of this book are not intended to be a substitute for professional medical or other healthcare advice, diagnosis or treatment and it is not the intention of the author to provide specific medical advice, but rather to provide readers with information about holistic approaches to maintaining and improving general health. Always seek the advice of your physician or other qualified healthcare provider with any questions you may have regarding any specific medical condition, medication or physical symptom. Never disregard professional medical advice or delay in seeking it because of something you have read in this book.

Index

A

A Natural Farm and Education Center, 72
acid reflux, 24, 107
acupressure, 27, 30–32
acupuncture, 8–11, 27–32
addictions, 11
alcohol, 18, 36, 38
Almond Milk recipe, 139
almonds, 85–87, 139
anti–inflammatory, 84, 123
antioxidants, 63, 100, 104
anxiety, 11, 88
apple cider vinegar, 43, 53, 99, 128, 150
apples, 54, 58, 63, 71, 73, 79, 147
apricot, 79
arthritis, 84
asthma, 11
astringent, 95–96
avocados, 71, 73, 82, 84, 87

B

baking, 113, 119, 121
banana, 52, 54–55, 61, 64, 73, 78, 134–135, 140, 143–144, 146
beans, 80
beets, 61, 79, 150
berries, 80, 98–100
beta carotene, 112
beverage recipes
    Almond Milk, 139
    Bittersweet Green Drink, 147
    Blood Builder Green Drink, 146
    Cashew Milk, 140
    Digestive Tonic Tea, 148
    Ginger Root Tea, 149
    Green Energy Booster, 145
    Green Smoothie #1, 143
    Green Smoothie #2, 144
    Spicy Lemonade, 142
bioflavonoids, 94
bitter, 25, 47, 61, 94, 108, 111
Bittersweet Green Drink recipe, 54, 147

blend, 53–54, 120

blood, 42, 61, 91, 100, 111

Blood Builder Green Drink
recipe, 55, 146

blood sugar, 78–80, 84

blueberries, 52, 62, 80, 143

body brushing, 40–44,
48–49

bran, 21

bread, 10, 22, 75, 78

breakfast, 20

breast feeding, 104

breath freshener, 108

breathing, 9, 27

bronchitis, 9

brown rice syrup, 139

buckwheat, 23, 151

burn fat, fat burning, 10, 84,
115

butterflies, 2–7, 100–101

C

cabbage, 58, 68

caffeine, 10

cake(s), 18, 21, 93

calcium, 85, 109

calorie(s), 17–18, 20, 83

candy, 75, 78

cantaloupe, 78

carbohydrates, 10, 22,
77–80, 83, 115

carminative, 104

carrots, 61, 63, 79

casein, 84

Cashew Milk recipe, 140

cashews, 87, 130, 137, 140

catnip tea, 25

cayenne pepper, 52, 142

celery, 47, 53, 128

cereals, 21, 75, 78, 151

chard, 59

chemicals, 14, 37, 107

cherries, 55, 80, 146

chia seeds, 52, 81, 137

child birth, 29

chlorophyll, 55, 61, 111

cholesterol, 81, 115

chrysalis, 3–4, 6

cinnamon, 136, 148

circulation, 40–44

citrus, 92–94

citrus zest, 93

cleansing, 34–56, 61, 93, 108

coconut, 115–121, 130, 134

coconut butter, 115, 120

coconut flour, 121

coconut milk, 120

coconut oil, 84, 115, 119, 121,
136, 138

coconut vinegar, 121

H

harvest, 58–73

headaches, 8, 28

healing, 8–11

health food store, 22, 25, 41, 46, 80, 87, 115

healthcare, 8–15, 27, 29–32

healthy eating, 58–153

healthy living, 2–32

healthy oils, 81–87, 115

heart, 42, 107

hemorrhoids, 32, 107

hemp oil, 84

hemp seeds, 82

herb(s), 13, 25, 70

herbicides, 34, 109

hesperidin, 94

high fructose corn syrup, 78, 80

holistic, 2–15, 24–32

honey, 25, 52, 78, 130, 135, 137–139, 142, 148–149

hormones, 8, 24–25, 76

hunger, 16, 20

hybridized, 94

I

ice cream, 91, 119

immune system, 41

indigestion, 104

infertility, 29

instar, 2

insulin resistance, 78

iridology, iris, 12–15, 34–39, 88

iron, 109

J

jam, 78

joint pains, joints, 11, 13, 43

juice fast, 38

K

kale, 58–59, 63, 66, 80, 152–153

Kale and Spinach Chips recipe, 153

ketchup, 75

ketoacidosis, 77

kidney stones, 37

kidneys, 35–38, 77

kitchen, 17–18, 34

kiwi, 64

L

Lake Meadow Naturals, 68
leafy tops, 60–61
legumes, 80
lemon, 52, 55–56, 80, 127, 129, 142, 145
lettuce, 18, 53, 58, 61, 80, 128
lifestyle, 2–88
limes, 71, 80, 134
limonene, 108
liver, 14, 24, 30, 35–38, 61, 93, 94, 108
Liver and Gallbladder Cleanser Salad recipe, 56, 129
Local Roots, 91
locally grown, 58–76, 90–114
low fat, 18, 77
lunch, 20, 58
lungs, 9
lymph, lymphatic system, 35–39, 42

M

macaroons, 121
macronutrients, 77
magnesium, 112
manganese, 96, 100, 112, 123
Mango Lime Sorbet recipe, 134
mango(es), 58, 78, 90–91, 134

manifest, 7
marinades, 121
meal(s), 14, 16–18, 20, 22–24, 34, 47, 85, 104, 115
meat, 17, 76
meat substitutes, 75
meditation, 4
Medjool dates, 136
medium chain triglycerides, 115
meridian(s), 8
metabolism, 22
metamorphosis, 2–7
millet, 23, 79–80, 151
minerals, 21, 61–62, 85, 91, 96, 100, 104, 107–108, 112, 115, 120
mood disorders, 84
morning sickness, 29–30
mucilage, 105, 107, 133
mulberries, 68
multivitamin, 62
muscles, 27, 43, 77

N

nausea, 29–32
neck, 27, 42
nicotine, 10
non-perishable, 22

CPSIA information can be obtained
at www.ICGtesting.com
Printed in the USA
LVHW01s0820250817
546344LV00004B/6/P